## Praise for *Sonny*

'Compelling reading, Kennaway explores the interlinked relationships between a young disabled boy, his mother and himself with unflinching honesty, asking searching questions most wouldn't dare with hilarious and heart-wrenching results. As he confronts his own challenges facing the world of disability, he takes the reader along on his journey into the life and interior world of Sonny, a young man with complex needs. The profound questions Kennaway poses and conclusions he reaches cover territory few others are brave enough to explore... Very moving.'

*Katie Glass*

'*Sonny* is a deeply moving portrait of a family battling Sonny's unimaginable physical and mental challenges with bravery, warmth and acceptance, endless resilience and ingenuity, but above all, love. An emotional rollercoaster that never lets up. Written with Guy Kennaway's trademark eye for detail and sense of humour, the prose never pulls its punches, but it pulls you into a warm embrace too. Like the best books, it is both heartbreaking and heartwarming: raw, tender and searingly honest. Unforgettable.'

*Veronica Henry*

'There are other books in which someone finds their humanity through contact with those living on the brink of existence, but none of them are as funny, as rakingly self-exposing, or as truthful as this one.'

*Nicola Shulman*

'This is such a brave book. Not for the faint hearted, Guy against all odds, enters into this extreme and affecting area of intense social care, and in what has become his leitmotif, regards it with his gimlet eye combining a mixture of empathy, sympathy, bewilderment and dazzling black humour.'

*Sarah-Jane Lovett*

'Guy Kennaway's extraordinary account of his friendship with a family and their son is much more than a story of caring for a disabled child. Guy confronts his own humanity head on. Guy is all too human, and *Sonny* is often hilarious as Guy struggles to put his own desires first. But even Guy cannot escape the pull of Sonny and his family, leading to a radical rethinking of what it means to be one person among others, sharing space and caring for each other.'

*Nicholas Blincoe*

'This book tells the story of the batteries that keep us going: undying belief, the love of a mother, and the strength of bearing witness to those with a much more difficult existence than our own. Guy's writing is more real and exposing than anything I've ever read on disability. Sonny reminds us that we are not separated by the things that make us different, we are separated when we turn away from each other.'

*Rebecca Achieng Ajulu-Bushell*

Guy Kennaway was born in London and educated at Edinburgh University. He writes comic fiction and memoir. 'In all my work I like to be tender and funny, finding and writing about people who have been overlooked or dismissed.' He lives in Jamaica and Somerset. *Sonny* is his tenth book.

### Also by Guy Kennaway
*One People*
*Sunbathing Naked*
*Bird Brain*
*Time To Go*
*The Accidental Collector*
(Winner of Bollinger Everyman Wodehouse Prize for Comic Fiction)
*Foot Notes*
*Good Scammer*

## Praise for Guy Kennaway's earlier books

ONE PEOPLE

'Humorous from beginning to end, this is an ideal stress reliever... This year's funniest novel.'

*GQ Magazine*

BIRD BRAIN

'A wonderfully astute satire with full confidence in its own eccentricity... Ripe, rich, fun, this is a beautifully turned story, good to the very last drop.'

*Sunday Times*

TIME TO GO

'This is such an extraordinary book. It's bracingly honest, blisteringly funny, and then it knocks you sideways with its sadness and straightens you up with its good sense. Bit of a rollercoaster, really.'

*Deborah Moggach*

GOOD SCAMMER

'Wonderfully entertaining and surprisingly profound.'

*John Williams in Mail on Sunday*

# SONNY
## Love with no limit

GUY KENNAWAY

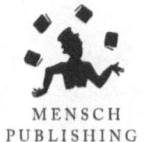

MENSCH
PUBLISHING

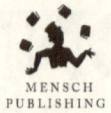

MENSCH
PUBLISHING

Mensch Publishing,

51 Northchurch Road,
London N1 4EE, United Kingdom

First published in Great Britain 2026

Copyright © Guy Kennaway 2026

Guy Kennaway has asserted his right under the Copyright, Designs and
Patents Act, 1988, to be identified as Author of this work

All rights reserved. No part of this publication may be reproduced or
transmitted in any form or by any means, electronic or mechanical,
including photocopying, recording, or any information storage or retrieval
system, without prior permission in writing from the publishers

A catalogue record for this book is available from the British Library

ISBN:
978-1-912914-86-9 (paperback)
978-1-912914-87-6 (eBook)

Typeset by Langscape
www.langscape.com

# Contents

| | | |
|---|---|---|
| 1. | The end | 1 |
| 2. | Glitter in her heart | 5 |
| 3. | Dying to meet you | 9 |
| 4. | Learning Sonny | 15 |
| 5. | Far from the Tree | 20 |
| 6. | Here, tonight | 24 |
| 7. | Into sync | 28 |
| 8. | An empty field and a few bystanders | 36 |
| 9. | The advocate | 40 |
| 10. | Formula | 50 |
| 11. | Room of Broken Things | 54 |
| 12. | A flash of colour | 57 |
| 13. | Express joy | 64 |
| 14. | Eye-Gaze | 72 |
| 15. | Relationship history | 90 |
| 16. | I couldn't explain how | 101 |
| 17. | Brutal environment | 111 |
| 18. | You'll never walk alone | 117 |
| 19. | A woman at an old wooden desk | 123 |
| 20. | The cot, the bedding, the rattles, the bottles | 127 |
| 21. | Blow torch and matches | 132 |
| 22. | Bliss amongst the crowd | 140 |
| 23. | Stuttering and failing | 146 |
| 24. | Random bunch of losers | 148 |
| 25. | It's strange | 154 |

| | | |
|---|---|---|
| 26. | Tell Them You Love Me | 156 |
| 27. | The Telepathy Tapes | 167 |
| 28. | Lifting the bread | 170 |
| 29. | Ticketing services | 175 |
| 30. | In the holidays I went skating | 179 |
| 31. | Heavy | 182 |
| 32. | Shark's head socks | 185 |
| 33. | Test results | 191 |
| 34. | Fixture | 199 |
| 35. | Sprinkles and whipped cream | 204 |
| 36. | XXXXL | 206 |
| 37. | Touchline village | 209 |
| 38. | Second half | 213 |
| 39. | Sapling | 217 |
| 40. | Barnsey | 220 |
| 41. | The beautiful game | 223 |
| 42. | The beginning | 226 |
| 43. | Secret place | 229 |
| Acknowledgements | | 231 |

# Disclaimer

The events in this book all happened, though not always in the sequence depicted. Time has been concertinaed to make the story readable and recollections, as the lady said, may vary. You might call it the varnished truth.

# 1

## The end

An electronic beep began to sound in stop-start traffic driving south through Spaghetti Junction.

'Is that the van or Sonny?' I asked from the passenger seat.

'Battery on the ventilator,' Andrea said, focused on the road, hands at ten to two. She was a trained ambulance driver and took the business of piloting the minibus seriously.

Maff stood up in the back, gave Sonny's hand a squeeze, and started digging through the bags while the beeping persisted.

'Can you see it?' Andrea said without glancing back.

Maff grunted and clipped open another case, found a battery, looked at it and put it back down. He started to go through the first suitcase again. We had left Liverpool in a hurry, at my urging, and could easily have left some of Sonny's equipment behind either in his hotel room or reception or on the pavement. There was just so much of it to keep track of. The flight cases, motorised chairs, oxygen cylinders and cardboard boxes of medical equipment made us look like a camera crew. Sonny, in his high and heavy chair, was the centre of it all: the camera, or was he the dozing director, swaddled in blankets and scarves, sunk in thought?

Maff started pulling clothes from a suitcase. It had been my idea, the trip to Liverpool. Sonny didn't usually venture far from his house. Needing a ventilator, monitoring machines and two carers made mobility tricky. I had dragged them all hundreds of miles north for a football match. And now we had mislaid the back-up battery. And as it turned out, that was a serious mistake.

'How long till it runs out?' I asked.

'We have seven minutes,' Andrea said. The dashboard clock said *16:06*. The ventilator had seven minutes of power, after which Sonny would stop getting air into his lungs, because he was unable to breathe without mechanical help. He lived a battery away from death.

I turned to look at Sonny in his chariot, swathed in Liverpool Football Club scarf and strip.

'Seven minutes to find the battery or get to mains electricity?' I asked.

'Yes,' said Maff.

Andrea said, 'Six. How far is the next service station?'

I looked on my phone. '*23* miles. Frankley.' The clock said *16:08*. The ventilator beeped.

## The end

Rain fell out of a filthy cloud, through the dusk and onto the windscreen. Ahead of us, a long snake of brake lights which oozed on and off was smeared across the glass by the wipers. In this traffic it would be forty minutes to Frankley. Across an old meadow criss-crossed with horse tape I saw the lights of a handful of houses. If we pulled onto the hard shoulder we could climb the Armco and carry Sonny across the field. He was a sixteen-year-old lad, and we'd have to take the ventilator, battery charger, suction pump, battery and a box of catheters. We'd leave the wheelchair behind. I had trouble enough getting that hulking thing over the lip of the hotel lift which was three millimetres high. Its little grey wheels would sink into that sodden turf. It was the stuff of a slow burning nightmare: pushing Sonny over a bog towards a strange house in failing light.

The van drew to a halt in the traffic. The beeps increased in volume, the gaps between them shortened. They were probably trying to be helpful, attracting the attention of a dozing carer, but they weren't.

I turned to Sonny and felt for his soft and comforting hand. He was imperturbable; silent and motionless, he accepted his fate. Which did not look promising.

'Traffic's bad,' said Andrea, eyes on the road. 'We could do with a blue flashing light.' Andrea had been a lead paramedic for nineteen years, including three-and-a-half years of training, but that was before Sonny was born.

'Maff,' said Andrea.

Maff grunted as he emptied out another suitcase. I swallowed; we were only in this situation because of my over-ambitious plan to drag Sonny across the country, when getting him from his bed to his school twelve miles away was a serious undertaking for three people.

The beeping morphed into a single painful note that burned a hole in my temple. The dashboard clock said *16.14*. The ventilator was about to stop. Give up the ghost. Literally. Andrea remained calm and focused on the road ahead, Maff was mumbling in the back. I had seen both retain their cool in medical crises with Sonny in the past, but this scared me. I turned to Sonny and gave him an encouraging smile. His oxygen level would now be well below the required 97%. He closed his eyes.

I said, 'What are we going to do?'

And the beeping abruptly ceased.

2

## Glitter in her heart

It was on a warm and dry September night, the kind of evening that made you feel how glorious the long soft summers of Somerset are, that I chanced upon Andrea. She was at the Hearthworks' party, standing under a festoon of coloured bulbs, a glass in her hand and a *1000*-watt smile on her face.

Hearthworks was the company of pirates and riggers who toured the music festivals with their yurts and tipis, honing their partying skills over the summer and giving them full rein at their end of season shindig – a legendary social event in Glastonbury, itself the global centre of excellence for good times.

Andrea was cherubic, in her mid-forties with striking blue eyes, glitter on her bonny cheeks and also, apparently, in her heart. Radiating kindness and naughtiness, she drew me in and pushed me away with perfect timing and a peal of laughter just engaging enough to keep me interested but to give me no real prospect of romantic hope. She was that social delight: a top-of-the-line flirt. After that evening, I didn't see her for a year, and then found her the following September, once again at the Hearthworks' staff junket. She stood in the same spot, under the same festoon of coloured bulbs.

Glastonbury is a small world and so there was something of the fairytale about her mysterious annual appearance. I asked her where she went for the rest of the year. She said her family kept her busy. She had four children, she said, and she mentioned that one required a lot of looking after. 'I don't get out much,' she smiled.

I asked her to come for lunch.

She said she was married.

I said, 'that doesn't stop you eating, surely?'

At lunch, months later, she showed me two photographs of Sonny and, as I listened to her, I understood the fairytale that she lived in. It was the one about a queen with a prince who wouldn't wake up.

I said, 'What's wrong with him?'

'Nothing,' she said. 'It's how he is.'

I thought, *I'm dealing with a nutter*. 'But what about the wheelchair and tubes?' I asked. 'Does he have a disease?'

'He has no diagnosis,' she said, 'but dystonia has been mentioned. We have had two years of genetic testing, and nothing has been found.' I went in for my first interview.

It wasn't a birth accident, that much I established. Birth accidents were easier for me, because then I could blame someone. It was definitely hereditary, or rather Sonny arrived on earth the way he was. But even after fourteen years, he had not had a diagnosis. Andrea was insistent on this. They couldn't get to the bottom of the problem.

But on one thing Andrea was clear: the half-light Sonny was living in was most definitely a dawn, a slow dawn, admittedly, but the sun on the horizon was rising, not setting.

'Can Sonny talk?' I asked.

'Not yet,' Andrea smiled. I took that to mean he struggled with words, but was improving.

I looked again at the photograph on her phone. 'All illness is difficult for me,' I said, 'but this kind of thing freaks me out.' I topped up our wine glasses. 'I fancy I'm pretty socially skilled,' I boasted modestly, 'and that you could put me down almost anywhere, from a socialite's dinner party in Belgravia to a bar in downtown Kingston, Jamaica, and I would know how to act, what to say, how to read the room, you know, deal with it, whatever came up ...but,' I swallowed a gulp, 'I never know what to say or do when I am with people like him.'

'He's called Sonny,' said Andrea.

'I don't know whether to try and talk, to just smile, to shake their hand, to bend down, or to ignore them and carry on. I don't even know whether to look at youngsters in wheelchairs when I pass them on the pavement. I mean, is that staring? What am I meant to do? So I just walk quickly by pretending not to see them.'

'Not that,' she said quietly.

'Right,' I said, 'I just don't know.'

'Lots of my friends feel the same way, I think,' she said. 'They are awkward, and I can see them struggling.'

'Is there a book I can read to tell me how to act, how to communicate?' I asked.

'There isn't a book,' she said.

'Maybe I could write one,' I said. 'For Sonny. A user's manual. With him, of course.'

She looked at me, and tipped her head to one side while she thought about this. 'Maybe you should,' she said.

'Will he help me? I mean, would he like me to?' I was imagining that I would basically be jotting down the world according to Sonny, in between having cups of tea and chats with Andrea.

'I will ask him,' she said.

There. He obviously *could* talk. Probably just a bit slowly or with a stammer. This book would be a doddle, and after having a good prowl around Amazon's top twenty books about disability, I realised I was writing into a marketing niche that not many other authors had noticed. Talk about falling off a log. How many disabled kids were there? You saw them everywhere these days. If every family bought two copies I'd hit paydirt.

'See what he says,' I said. 'Tell him about my other work.'

'I think it's a very good idea,' she said.

3

**Dying to meet you**

I approached the Thompson home in Frome, Somerset, and peered through the glazed front door at a barking terrier turning tight circles on the doormat. Andrea let me in, led me past racks of children's shoes, and into the kitchen.

'Would you like to meet Sonny?' she asked, looking at me with those pale bluey-green, almost turquoise eyes, full of fun and light. 'Come on, he's dying to meet you.'

I nodded, pulling on a smile. What had I got myself into it? I was feeling grim. This was scary. I felt like making an excuse and leaving. I even had one ready: earache, which I had been encouraging by prodding with my fingernail all morning.

By sheer force of personality, Andrea pulled me behind her through the clean but cluttered sitting room. We passed a woman with a bag at her feet and her head in a phone who ignored us. On we went through a pair of unpainted double doors and into a bedroom attached to the back of the house with a view out onto a tiered garden going up the hill. I knew this extension had been constructed just for Sonny, because getting him upstairs had got too difficult.

Sonny lay on his back on a massage table in the middle of the room. He had a head of curly amber hair, pale smooth skin and big brown eyes that roamed across me. They possessed his mother's kindness, and also what seemed to be fear. He was naked except for a towel over his tummy that went down to his knees.

'He's about to have his massage. Aren't you?' Andrea said. That explained the woman in the chair checking her phone.

I was introduced to Zoe, a tall, attractive young woman who was hovering sympathetically around Sonny. She was one of his carers, a part of a thing called the care package, which was help given to Sonny by the State. Once the lady in the chair and Zoe were squeezed in beside the bed I could see it came at a cost of personal privacy.

Lying on my back naked under a towel was not how I would like to meet someone for the first time.

'Hello,' I said.

Sonny didn't reply with any words or sounds. I was not sure if this was because he couldn't or because he didn't want to. His eyebrows moved, his eyes opened wider, and he looked up at the ceiling behind him. I had absolutely no idea what he was communicating. It could have been:

*Hello, how are you? Good to meet you.*

Or

*Can you please get out of here, I'm naked under this towel and it's weird meeting a stranger right now.* Which is what I would be thinking.

Andrea said, 'He's pleased to see you, aren't you Sonny?'

I thought, *where did she get that from?* Was there some pheromonic exchange between their skins that I was not sensing?

'This is Guy, I told you about him.'

His eyes opened wide again, and moved roughly in my direction. I searched them for meaning. I now realised that my assumption had been incorrect. He couldn't talk. He was fourteen years old, with his skin as soft and pink as a six-month old baby. I haven't mentioned the first thing I noticed: a ribbed translucent pipe going into a valve in the front of his throat. That was the ventilator which provided the air for him to live.

'He says hello,' Andrea said.

I said, 'Hello Sonny, I am a writer of books. I have written a book about my mum, and another book about walking across Britain, and even an award-winning comedy about the London art world, and I would like to write a book about you. I want to tell your story.'

His eyes moved around the ceiling, then passed over me. It was hard to tell what he took in. His eyebrows raised, stayed up and then lowered.

'He likes that,' Andrea said, standing at his head looking down at him. 'Let's put your glasses on,' she said, producing a pair with quite thick glass in fashionable tortoiseshell frames. They weren't the game changer I hoped for. His eyes still moved round the room, pausing momentarily on me and sweeping on across the shelves of toys and floor cabinet of medical equipment.

I stood there. I didn't know what to say.

Seeing a football scarf by the bed, I tried, 'I see you support Liverpool.'

Ok. Definitely saw some energy there. His eyes widened and his eyebrows moved.

'So do I. Did you see the game last night?'

A delicate wrinkling of his forehead. And a downwards micro shrug of his shoulders. I knew he had. We had been beaten by Burnley *0-1*. I had turned the TV off after forty miserable minutes and made myself a sandwich of beef, mayo, ham and cheese on white to take the pain away.

'He watches every game,' Andrea said. 'Him and Maff. They were gutted.' I hadn't met Maff, Andrea's husband and Sonny's father. He was at work in Bath, in a studio where he restored antique furniture.

'Bad season, yeah?'

Wrinkled forehead.

'It's because we lost Van Dijk,' I said.

His eyes roamed the room. I turned to see a poster of Virgil Van Dijk, the Liverpool defender, ball imperiously at his feet, about to make a raking pass out of defence to our lads up front. Van Dijk had been out for six weeks with a leg injury.

'It's all gone tits up since we lost him,' I said.

Was that a smile? I couldn't tell, but I definitely thought I was through to Sonny.

'I think he needs a clear,' Andrea said. 'Do you want to?' she said to him, looking over his head from behind where he lay. 'Or you don't want to?'

There was a rustle of action. Andrea placed her hands on his chest and pressed so hard it looked injurious to me. His ribs bent deep into his lungs. They seemed oddly soft, like rubber. Then she took a clear plastic straw from the pack by the table, attached it to a transparent rubber tube, removed the ribbed tube from the plastic valve in his throat, and

slid the straw into the hole and down into his lungs to a depth of about twelve inches. It was exceedingly uncomfortable to watch, forget experience, though as Sonny could not move or make any noise it was hard to know how painful it was for him. Andrea leant over him and turned on a pump. I heard it draining some fluid. She then pulled it out and reattached the thick breathing pipe.

## Sonny

Christ. *Do you want to? You don't want to?* That was his mum asking. That meant Andrea was having trouble distinguishing a yes from a no. And she had fourteen years of practice speaking to him. Yet after that short confusion I started believing that Andrea, and Zoe for that matter, were communicating with him. But I couldn't quite see how.

## 4

## **Learning Sonny**

Learning Sonny was going to be a lot trickier than I thought. He couldn't speak, or move anything except his eyes, face and shoulders. That was quite a limited vocabulary.

Andrea smiled brightly as she used another suction machine to remove goo that was dripping out of the corner of Sonny's mouth. Her other hand ruffled his auburn hair and as she pulled out the pipe she bent to kiss his forehead. While she worked she was totally focused on watching him, a glow of pride in her cheeky smile. There was no doubt, no sadness, no defeat and no pain on her face or in her body language. I suspect I was ashen and stiff, as I stood there frozen with shock.

'I don't think we are going to win the premiership this year,' I managed to say, when his pit stop was over.

A downward tilt of the edge of his eyes which slightly saddened his angelic face. That was a NO. Definitely. Or was it an admonishing 'Oh yes we are!'

'That's a no, isn't it?' I queried.

A barely perceptible smile, which forced a dribble of saliva from the corner of his mouth.

'Right, I think I'm picking this up. Let's try this: do we want Man U to win the League?'

Extreme downward slant of eyes. Clear dread in irises.

'Right,' I said. 'We definitely have contact. Great.' I beamed a smile at him, and Andrea looked from me to Sonny and back again, nodding and smiling.

'Thank god for that,' I didn't say.

'Have you ever been to a Liverpool game?' I asked.

'No,' Andrea answered. I was looking at Sonny. He appeared to me as though he was listening, his expression not yet formed.

'That would be a good thing for us to do,' I said brightly. 'I've been to Anfield a few times,' I told him. 'That would be a trip.'

Andrea said, 'We have thought about it but it's very difficult. Well, impossible really. Hotels are tricky because he has to have his lungs suctioned every fifteen minutes, so it means we have to do it ourselves or bring carers, which means more rooms.'

'He has that done to him through the night as well?'

'He sleeps through suctioning him, rolling him, if you're gentle. You can move him on to his side and change him and he'll stay asleep. But a night away is a challenge. There's the chair and pump pack and extra batteries and the carer. Maybe me and Maff could do it together, but it's a bit of an impossibility for both of us to get away because of the other kids.'

'Of course.'

Sonny's massage was about to commence. They had the time booked.

I said, 'I've got to go now.' I wondered, how often had he heard people say that? Sonny could never leave. It wasn't something he would say, or could say. He had to wait for others to leave.

'But I will come back, and I will spend time with you and I will stay longer next time. I just wanted to say hello.'

Zoe and Andrea had left the room to go about other tasks, and we were alone for the first time. I stepped closer. 'I can't tell you what people will make of our book, but I will write it as best I can and be truthful. All right?'

I looked into his face.

I was no longer looking for words, but there was so little to go on in terms of expression and eye movement. Language was an ability that Sonny could not master, like mobility, like breathing for goodness sake.

I said goodbye, left the bustle and commotion of the house, got into my car and put my forehead on the steering wheel. I thought, *what have I got myself into? Why am I doing this?* I have basically promised Sonny I'm going to write his story.

But the problem was – well there were so many problems, where to start? The MAIN problem was that he terrified me. Lying there, unable to move anything except his eyes and the skin on his face, and then not apparently in total control of them, not to mention being unable to breathe without that pipe and pump. I was involved with a subject that scared me, terrified me: disability. I did a feelings check: guilt; fear; pain; bottomless sadness about a life not lived.

Sonny was up there in the top three of my very worst fears. He was the worst-case scenario incarnate. I used to sweat as my children came to parturition, praying please god don't let the baby emerge – well I would now say *like Sonny* – and here I was. Involved with him for months, maybe years.

I didn't know any disabled people.

A fist tightened in my chest at the thought of being in proximity to disability. It was defending my heart from infection. My strategy of dealing with the lame and needy was to ignore and avoid them. I lived my life carving a path around anything I found difficult, and then covering my tracks with bullshit.

Driving home over the Mendip plateau and then into the Glastonbury valley, seeing the Tor on its grassy cone appear out the mist, I remembered where I had seen a group of people like Sonny before: at football matches. When I watched televised football I saw spectators in wheelchairs with football scarves lining the touchline of big matches. Fans. Disabled. In the front row. I particularly recalled noticing them when I was a boy. The reason it was so memorable was because people like Sonny were otherwise invisible in my 1960s and 70s childhood. I really cannot remember ever seeing a disabled child except for the sinister statue of the boy with calipers on Hampstead High Street which was a charity collection box outside the greengrocers. I wonder if there was a disabled child hidden from the uncaring world in an upstairs room who had prompted their parents to put out the plaster beggar. Apart from that, the only others I saw were at the football, where they were very much on display. I will be honest: I didn't like seeing them. They freaked me out. There, I've said it.

As I neared my home, a plan started coming together in my mind. My thoughts returned to the football pitch. I was thinking about a particular match: the European Cup Final, at the Ataturk Olympic Stadium, Istanbul (the location of another of Liverpool's European triumphs in 2005), on Saturday 29th May 2021. About two months away. Liverpool were not only going to be there, but were going to win it, as they had the year before. I wanted to be in the crowd to enjoy the triumph. But tickets were impossible to get. Impossible. I had already tried and failed, and I had some good connections with the club. But that was before, that was before I was taking Sonny. How could they possibly refuse him, and his carer (me, for that day) a ticket? And what a seat. Right at the front, within talking distance of the gods on the pitch.

I was warming to the project. I looked forward to telling Sonny we were going to Istanbul, and should start making plans.

## 5

## Far from the Tree

I went onto the laptop I am typing this on, opened Amazon in Safari and looked for books about disability. I was pleased to see a meagre selection. To cheer myself up, I bought the one that looked most dire. Self-published and featuring a cover with a sugary picture of a child with no evident disability, it was called *The Child Who Spoke with Her Eyes*. When it turned up it had the unpromising density of a self-published book. *The Child Who Spoke with Her Eyes* was written by a courageous woman about her daughter, born in the mid-sixties, in the long dark era for disabled kids and their parents. It was brave but sugar-dipped. She swerved every painful truth. But also, I noticed another feature of her narrative, which chilled me. It was dismally stagnant, because no matter what the mum tried with her daughter, no progress was ever made, at least not in the direction she longed for it to go. The programme to get the girl to feed herself, which started so optimistically with the introduction of a spoon on page *21*, was still showing no results with food all over the floor and an exhausted mum on page *116*. Every writer knew that development of plot and character was what made a book readable. The little girl in the book didn't have a narrative arc, or character development. How could she? It was like describing a photograph, and nothing else. It made for tough reading. And now this challenge was mine.

A second book had turned up and was altogether different. It dealt almost exclusively with painful truths. Called *Far from the Tree*, it was an astonishing compendium of the lives of weird kids, their parents and their siblings. Painful, uplifting, and exhaustive, the writer, a chap called Andrew Solomon, interviewed hundreds of parents like Maff and Andrea and dug into scores of academic papers for some conclusions. For anyone with a connection to anyone like Sonny, I cannot recommend reading chapters 1 and 7 strongly enough.

It was from *Far from the Tree* (FFTT) that I learnt that SMD – Severe Multiple Disabilities – was the correct description of Sonny's medical condition. Clever as Solomon was, I discovered that many of the experts on SMD patients and their families were ill-informed. Apparently, parents of SMD children have what psychologists call 'Chronic Sorrow'. Those who don't exhibit it are seen as over-compensating to disguise rage, guilt and overpowering wishes to harm their child. I typed that sentence almost verbatim from FFTT, which was itself quoting the counsellor Simon Olshansky. I know nothing of Olshansky except that he definitely hadn't met Andrea or Maff. And he should.

SMD is a shorthand description rather than a medical diagnosis, which is what everyone I spoke to about Sonny seemed to want. Apart from Andrea and Maff, that is.

One particular passage I had read during my research stuck in my mind. It said that *no* diagnosis of a sick child was the most difficult of all diagnoses for parents to deal with. 'Once the course is clear,' wrote Solomon, 'most people can accept it. Syndromes associated with dire prospects are borne more nobly than those of which little is understood.' I have googled dystonia as Andrea had mentioned it. It was a neurological movement disorder that usually made people shake and shudder (which Sonny didn't do). Life expectancy of a dystonia patient was low.

To accept and to announce to the world that Sonny had dystonia, or even something else, would possibly place Andrea and Maff in an easier position for society to manage. We would all say it's dystonia. It would be known that Sonny may well not make it to twenty-five. That would alter my reaction to the situation. But if you heard Maff or Andrea talk about the future, for instance the plan for Sonny to go to college, you'd get the impression Sonny was going to live into ripe old age.

It was not long after I met Sonny for the first time that I was having a drink with Andrea and friends, and talking about his non-verbal immobility.

A woman asked, 'What's wrong with Sonny?'

Andrea replied, 'Nothing.'

The woman looked a little confused, then embarrassed, and tried to change the subject. I guess she thought Andrea must have misunderstood the question or was simply bonkers, possibly driven mad by her incapacitated child.

But I nodded, knowingly, and smiled, because after only a few encounters with Sonny and Andrea I was already leaving the world I had lived in, in which disability was a scary thing to be kept far away, and touching down on Andrea and Sonny's planet where disability was the norm, where it was safe to approach, and was nothing to be frightened of.

## 6

### Here, tonight

I invited Andrea and Maff for dinner at my place. Andrea texted: *I think we may have found someone to cover from 7.30, meaning being to you around 8pm. Does that work?* (3 weeks in advance).

And she also texted a week later: *I'm so excited to be actually going out with Maff and to be spending time with you. Super excited. Would you like a contribution towards dinner?*

They turned up late, because there was a problem getting the new carer to do the catheter suction the way they wanted her to. The council had awarded Sonny's care package to a new company. The last company had a team of eighty staff looking after thirty kids. The new one had a staff of thirty to look after five children. I assumed this would dilute the number of carers but when I did the maths I discovered that the ratio remained the same. Zoe had moved company to stay with Sonny, but nearly all of his carers were now new to him.

Andrea had told me it was the first time in four years that she and Maff had managed an evening out together. I was expecting some awkwardness (because Sonny metaphorically hovered in the background as all the guests knew about our project), but the two of them lit up the room with joy and enthusiasm, and settled around the kitchen table to join in the conversation with the glee of a happy couple having their first dinner out together in four years. Both Maff and Andrea radiated a mischievous warmth. I liked Maff very much, and I could see the two of them, when you took everything into account, were miraculously and admirably in love. It's a well-known fact amongst the parents of disabled children that 97% of couples break up within five years of the birth.

The plan to flirt with and seduce Andrea was most definitely and happily axed.

I had been worried that the evening might have been a bit stilted, with my guests self-conscious. Sonny wasn't there, but he was there, and I knew how hard we, with the exception of Maff and Andrea, all found him to deal with. When I had described Sonny to my friends there was often an intake of breath. Most were sorry, some bewildered, and some were angry, I'm not sure why, I suspect because they were frightened of the thought of Sonny. One or two shook their heads and questioned why he was alive. One said 'maybe it would be better if he hadn't lived. You know, all round for everyone. I mean, what is his quality of life?'

I answered that that was what I was going to investigate in my book.

But I had read some of the writings of Judith Heumann, the pioneering disability rights campaigner in the USA, and she had posed this question to people with 'healthy normal' kids: *have you ever wished one of them had never been born?*

I need not have worried about my other guests at dinner. I think their main reaction to Andrea was surprise and delight. At various points in the evening, between sitting down to eat, standing around the log fire in rapid conversation, and pushing the kitchen table back so everyone could dance, I watched Andrea and Maff move amongst the company sprinkling happy dust over us.

At first I thought we all felt so good because we had the opportunity to be supportive of Maff and Andrea, without experiencing any of the actual pain of a close encounter with Sonny, with all its difficult and upsetting details. I had already recognised a propensity in people to give Andrea support from a safe distance. I watched guests attend closely to Andrea, offering her drink (which she refused as she wasn't a big drinker), cigarettes and kind conversation. She and Maff glowed with the attention. They were our night flowers: tropical jasmines which bloomed after dark and perfumed the moonlight.

I'm not sure what the evening was like for them, but it definitely made me feel wonderful. I was a towering humanitarian. All of us were carrying them, on their evening out. Nobody said anything to me, but we all knew that this was a special event for them, being out together without any responsibility beyond keeping their glasses full and having a good time. They brought with them to the party a sense of beauty and fun and a kind of lightness about life, which to an old cynic like me, worn down by cares, was welcome and indeed needed. They didn't say, *Look what we carry, and look how lightly we move,* but we thought it.

Watching as she leant towards the open fire to light a cigarette, it would have been reasonable to think *aren't we lucky we don't have THAT at home to worry about and take up all our time?*

But as she turned to look at the room, her pale blue eyes and easy smile spoke to us: *We are all lucky. All of us. You are, and Maff and I are, and even Sonny is. Never forget how lucky we all are, here, tonight, together.*

## 7

### Into sync

My next visit to Sonny was on a spring morning in *2021*. The pandemic had slowed the project. I drove the *15* miles from my house to Frome with dread like a lump of lead in my gut. Heavy and poisonous. If you came in to town from the direction I did, you went through some fairly deprived housing estates before dropping into the decidedly chi-chi streets on the hills of the mainly Victorian town. Frome has a reputation for being rather pleased with itself, even smug. This was totally deserved, in my opinion. Though I was feeling tight and uncharitable that bright morning.

When I arrived, Sonny was being showered and dressed behind the unpainted double doors of his suite. He had been given the day off school for this get-to-know-Guy session. School was, I think, a place where he went and spent time with other kids who have it particularly tough, kids like him. I made a note that I had to go and see what that was like but I dreaded going in case it was so upsetting it spoilt the strange harmony of Andrea's world.

Andrea was in the kitchen.

'All right,' she said into the phone, 'I'll pick them up from you, bring them here and you can pick her up from mine. I'll give her tea, and if you can take Talulah tomorrow to dance lessons and I will pick them both up and drop off Ali after the class.'

Andrea had a minibus to do all her picking up and dropping off with.

Zoe opened the doors, ushered me in, and went about her business sorting out medical paraphernalia and filling in paperwork. I found myself alone with Sonny, who was sitting up in a large, motorised wheelchair. His seat could be lowered and tilted automatically, but not by him of course. He wore a t-shirt, neckerchief, trousers and fancy socks with no shoes.

'Remember me?' I asked.

I sensed that he did.

You may well ask how I sensed that. Did he say anything? No, obviously. Did he give a look of recognition? No, actually. But I still thought he knew who I was. At the time, in the early days of our acquaintanceship, I had thrown myself into the project of believing in Sonny. I happily let myself be carried along on Andrea's burning certainty about his capacity to communicate. And it seemed to be working. I didn't allow doubts to cloud my judgement. I admit it, I wanted him to recognise me, I wanted him to interact with me.

## Sonny

When I tapped my pocket and realised I had left my notebook in the car I said, 'I've just got to nip out. I'll be right back,' and added, 'don't go away,' to see if he smiled.

He didn't smile. But that didn't dismay me. I thought, *Ah he wants to smile, but can't*, or, failing that, the fault in communication was mine and I hadn't quite done the joke well enough. But out at the car, as I felt into the door pocket for my notebook, I thought of another option: maybe my joke had been too tough, too cruel and had simply slayed the lad. Joking to him about never being able to move. How kind was that?

When I returned with my notes, I stood in the room and readjusted my settings, my internal linguistic and communication devices, to a higher sensitivity. I moved slowly and deliberately, kept my gaze on Sonny, and let my facial expressions pass over my face without haste. I even tried to start thinking slowly, to get into sync with Sonny.

I once saw a memorable bit of film of an earthquake rescue operation. I think it was in Italy. A block of flats had collapsed, and rescuers under spotlights were swarming over the rubble searching for survivors. Two big diggers stood to one side delicately picking up wreckage and pouring it into trucks. A man shouted out, and everyone fell silent. The digging stopped, the generator was turned off, the trucks cut their engines. This was so that they could listen for any faint noise from deep under the pile of the demolished building. Someone had heard a tapping under the hill of masonry, dust and twisted rebar.

## Into sync

Three hundred people stopped what they were doing and stood motionless. Everyone strained their ears. Not a cough. Not a whisper. This was life and death. And somewhere under them, in the dark, with the ceiling pressing his head and the water at his chest, Sonny had found a broken mug and was tapping on a pipe.

I was inching my way towards him through that mountain of broken concrete, shards of glass, and brick dust.

'I don't know if you can understand me, or understand even some of what I am saying,' I started, dropping my voice and talking slowly, 'but I'm going to proceed on the basis that you can. I guess that's what I would want if I were you. Look,' I said, now almost whispering, but enunciating clearly, 'I'm going to level with you. I only took this gig because I fancied your mum and didn't know she was married.'

Sonny's eyes had stopped roaming the ceiling and far wall and were fixed on me. Both of them. I heard the tap on the pipe.

'But I met your dad and really rate him and obviously shagging your mum is no longer an option.' Sonny held his stare. Was that a slight movement of his eyebrows? 'It did slightly remove the gloss from the project, I will be honest,' I told the lad. 'I did think about gently backing out. Yes, I did. Oh, you are sad. I can see you are sad. Well, here I still am, but frankly I am at a bit of a loss to see how I am going to do this.

'The truth is, my friend, you really scare me. I have never met anyone like you, and when I see kids like you I ... what do I do?

## Sonny

I look straight through you. I have a granddaughter called Lola. She is about to be five. She is a really friendly, outgoing, fun little girl. She loves skipping around, talking to strangers and making friends. I took her to the playground last year and saw a child in a wheelchair a bit like you and I saw his mum standing alone, apart from the other parents and nannies. It was in London, it was autumn and there were a lot of nannies grouped up on the dead leaves of the plane trees, and I pretended not to notice the child in the wheelchair and the mum, and I should have ... I wish I had ... I wish I had taken Lola over to say hello. But I was ... what? I was scared and embarrassed. When I was young, people used to say, "Don't Stare", but I think now that was just something they said to feel good about ignoring kids like you, excluding them. It's so stupid, but seems such a powerful force that stops me making contact. I guess it's fear of the unknown, though usually I am drawn to the unknown so it can't have been that ... in fact, the unknown has a magnetic appeal to me. Maybe it was fear of contagion, like some deep-rooted thing in my DNA to avoid illness. I don't know. Maybe just straight cowardice. I feel ashamed, Sonny,' I blushed, and felt tears of regret and pain pricking my eyes. 'Anyway, here I am now,' I shook my head slowly. 'I have a lot to learn, I guess.'

'How are you two getting on?' Andrea said as she and Zoe blasted through the door. I took out a handkerchief and pretended to blow my nose as I wiped my eyes. The two of them busied themselves with the terrifying pressing of his soft rib cage and attaching the pump. With a final suction of his mouth he was rearranged on his chair and the double doors to the sitting room were re-opened.

'What do you want to do, Sonny?' Andrea asked.

'I don't know,' I fantasised him saying, 'but can you get this weirdo out of my room?'

I said, 'May I touch your hand, Sonny?'

I think Andrea was about to answer, but I searched Sonny's face for a reply. I sensed a softness in his attitude. He had probably realised he was landed with me and had better make the best of it. Sentiments I expect he was all too familiar with.

'Thank you,' I said, and touched his hand, baby soft and motionless. I gave it a little squeeze and smiled.

'How come you're not at school?' I asked.

'He got the day off to spend some time with you,' Andrea said.

'Is that a good break?' I asked Sonny.

We peered into the oracle.

'Are you saying you would prefer to be at school?' Andrea said. I swallowed. 'Are you happy?' she asked him. 'Do you need more suction?' No discernible reply. Andrea took another tack. 'Are you happy to be at home?' Something changed on Sonny's face. 'Yes?' Pause, because we all felt there was something more to come out. Don't ask me how. It was the weirdest form of communication I have ever experienced. And I've lived with an adolescent child. It was a cross between a Ouija board and someone standing outside a double-glazed window in a high wind.

'Are you happy to be back at school tomorrow?' Andrea asked. 'Yes!' She cried. I joined in the general glee. The message had got through. But as I smiled and nodded I thought, hang on, I didn't see Sonny do anything. Was that reply entirely the creation of Zoe, Andrea and me? Was it a projection created by the three of us?

'He's such a loving, warm person,' Andrea said, ruffling his curls, which I must say looked very ruffleable and attractive. But I didn't think I was yet in a place with Sonny where it would be cool for me to touch his hair. 'No?' she questioned. Was she picking up micro cues I couldn't detect? Then Andrea said 'You don't want to go back to school! You're a hard ass. Yes!' And it was generally agreed that she'd hit the nail on the head, even if around the nail were quite a lot of deep indentations from hammer blows that had missed. It didn't matter.

'Do you want to talk to Guy about the story of PICU?' Andrea asked Sonny. It was decided he did, mainly because I had a feeling it was going to be important. PICU stood for Paediatric Intensive Care Unit. Andrea kicked off. 'Did you go in a helicopter or an ambulance?' We both stared at Sonny, willing him to give us a sign. The goodwill and encouragement in that room was almost intoxicating. Come on, Sonny, I was saying to myself. You can do this. Chopper or van? It had to be the chopper, or Andrea would never have mentioned it.

'Long think?' Andrea said.

We were now waiting for Sonny to say helicopter. You couldn't fault us for our optimism.

'He's closing down,' said Andrea.

'It must have been traumatic. I don't blame him. I blot out the difficult bits of my life,' I said.

'In *2012*,' Andrea then explained, 'Sonny got a cold that turned to pneumonia. Talulah had just been born when he was helicoptered to the Bristol Children's Hospital.'

## 8

## An empty field and a few bystanders

On the morning of the emergency, when Sonny was five years old, Andrea put her head around his bedroom door and sensed something was not quite right. She went closer: did he look pale and sound short of breath, or was it in her head? Ten years working in the ambulance service made Andrea cautious: it was well documented that mothers who were paramedics tended to catastrophise with their own family, so she didn't call 999. All morning she kept a watch on Sonny while looking after her new baby girl, Talulah, who she was at home with on maternity leave.

Sonny had a cold which had been getting worse. To stop secretions running from his nose and phlegm from his mouth, the doctor had proscribed patches called Hyoscine. Andrea didn't realise that while this drug dried Sonny's mouth and nose, it had allowed the liquid to accumulate in his lungs and fester into an infection. In those days Sonny breathed unaided by a ventilator.

Maff came home early. Together, they decided Sonny was breathing with his stomach rather than his chest. That meant he might not be getting enough air.

Despite her three years of formal training as a paramedic, Andrea still believed in super-alternative medicine. She practised Reiki on her patients, to me an inexplicable treatment, and proudly espoused what I considered magical medical treatments. I once asked her about a patch of psoriasis on my calf. She looked at it closely, and then said, 'I can help you with this. Right. First things first: what star sign are you?'

But on this occasion, she went super-conventional, and called her colleagues at ambulance control. She asked them to send a paramedic to check Sonny, because there was no monitoring equipment in the house. The ambulance turned up and the two paramedics hurried through the house with some cold March air. They opened their shoulder bags and checked Sonny's blood pressure, heartbeat and oxygen level. After a brief deliberation the paramedics informed Andrea and Maff that Sonny had to be airlifted by helicopter to hospital immediately. They stretchered Sonny to the ambulance and drove through the housing estate to the field opposite. Maff went with them. The chopper landed, loaded and disappeared into the sky leaving an empty field and a few bystanders.

Andrea organised for her mum to pick up her son Finn, seven, from school, gathered up Talulah and followed in the car. At the Bristol Children's Hospital, she parked and found Maff and Sonny in a holding ward next to A&E.

The doctors had interpreted Sonny's scans and X-Rays: both his lungs had collapsed and they couldn't get them back up. Sonny himself was ashen and unresponsive. The lung infection was rapidly worsening, and Sonny was on his way out.

The panic Andrea had been keeping locked in a box with a determined professional calm started banging at the lid. She and Maff were taken through the Intensive Care Unit where an alarming array of ailing sick and dying children lay. Amongst them, Sonny was motionless on a ventilator, under a web of tubes and wires. Nasal for air, chest for heart rate, finger for oxygen, and tummy for feeding. He had had the feeding tube in for over a year, since feeding him by mouth had turned out to be impossible. His swallow reflex was so weak Andrea and Maff had sometimes spent ten hours spooning a single meal into him.

I'll repeat that.

They sometimes spent ten hours spooning a single meal into him.

The doctors wanted a conversation.

'I'm afraid you need to prepare yourselves for the worst,' the paediatrician told Andrea, who was holding Talulah asleep in her arms. She and Maff looked down at Sonny's cherubic face, glabrous skin and curls.

'You probably need some rest,' the doctor said. 'If you want to go home, we will call if anything happens.'

Andrea held her son's hand and felt Maff's arm tighten around her shoulders.

She shook her head. 'I'll be staying here, until we take him home,' she said.

## 9

## The advocate

'How long was he in for?' I asked, perching on the bed, noticing that Sonny did not move his feet to give me more room.

'We spent *307* days at that place, mainly with Sonny in the Intensive Care Unit. He was nasally ventilated because his breathing wasn't strong enough. The plan was to wean him off it.'

'So up to five-years-old, he was breathing on his own?'

'Yes,' said Andrea. That was tough to hear, because it established for the first time with Andrea that there was a decline in health going on, a fact which, for I think excellent reasons, had never been mentioned before.

'Do you need suction?' Andrea asked Sonny. His eyebrows rose into a point over his nose in what was clearly a pained expression. Andrea positioned her palms on his chest and pressed about six times. Hard. Every impulse in me shouted "Stop! He's a child!" It was shocking how violent it seemed, and how deeply his ribs bent inwards. Then she changed the pipes in the hole in his throat, turned on the pump and cleared the liquid. Then she reconnected the ventilator and ran the dentist style suction pipe around his mouth and under his tongue. Within four minutes he was back sitting in his chair with his neckerchief around his neck.

'He came out of hospital on a ventilator,' Andrea said. So Sonny had been like this for nearly ten years? That was good. That was a good sign, I told myself. That's a positive.

'He had been really struggling with breathing nasally. And he had the tracheostomy in August *2012* while in PICU.' I guessed that was the valve in his neck.

'We had to fight to get you home, didn't we?' Andrea kissed Sonny on the forehead. 'The hospital had pretty much surrendered.'

Sonny was in critical care in Bristol. Andrea and Maff stayed in accommodation beside the hospital, along with Talulah, with Finn visiting. The place they stayed was a hostel for the family of sick children paid for by McDonald's Restaurants, a corporation that Andrea, as a committed vegetarian, would usually have avoided. But she was on a mission. And her mission was Sonny. And nothing could get in the way of that.

When Sonny stabilised in the Intensive Care Unit he had the tracheostomy fitted. They made a hole in the front of his neck into his windpipe and inserted a plastic fitting into which they could clip the ribbed air pipe. Sonny was six months in critical care. That's *180* days and nights when he could have died at any time. Finn was schooled in the hospital, where they had a room and teachers for children in his position; children whose sick siblings were forcing compromises on their upbringing. Talulah was with Andrea and Maff in the waiting area of the Unit. She took her first steps using a saline drip for support.

Sonny's parents enjoyed good relationships with the doctor, but Sonny himself was a 'no go' for the consultant, to use Andrea's words. The man didn't believe Sonny would thrive or even survive outside the Intensive Care Unit of the Bristol Children's Hospital. This disagreement escalated until Sonny's case was taken to the Ethics Board of the NHS which would decide whether or not it was viable for him to go home. Whether, basically, he had enough quality of life to be allowed to go home and live. Naturally, Andrea was convinced he did. The case turned on whether he could thrive on the day ventilator, which was mobile, battery-powered and produced cold, non-humidified air. The NHS decreed that any patient who had to have a constant supply of mains electricity to survive could not be defined as thriving.

Sonny was given an advocate to represent his interests. Strange, considering he already had Andrea, but not for the first or the last time, the authorities did not automatically believe that his parents were acting in Sonny's best interest.

It was an insulting proposition, but maybe necessary in a world where not all parents were like Andrea and Maff.

'We spent days and weeks in the parents' room at the ICU,' Maff told me. He had come home from work and joined in the conversation before going to pick up the girls. 'Drama,' he said, kissing Sonny, murmuring to him and squeezing his hand. 'So much tragedy. It was normal to walk through the unit and see a child with an open chest, totally open.'

'Did you get to know the other parents?'

'Lots of them,' said Maff. 'So many families coming in and out. All the tragedy going on around us when their children died. Like us, they were waiting, and unlike us they went home, sometimes for good reasons, taking their child with them, and sometimes not ...'

Andrea felt the mood sag and did two of her favourite things: lift the vibe and involve Sonny.

'Sonny enjoyed the activity of the ICU. Didn't you? All the comings and goings, all the people saying hello to him.'

'But you couldn't leave?'

'They wouldn't let us,' Andrea said.

*The NHS basically wanted to just let him die,* I thought to myself. That would not have been a workable strategy with a mum like Andrea.

'They said he couldn't be looked after properly at home,' she said. 'So we fought them all the way to the NHS ethics committee.

'The people who make all those horrible life and death decisions,' I said.

'Yes,' Andrea replied.

Andrea and Maff made sure they were involved in making representations about the decision to keep Sonny in hospital, and after 307 days they overturned the NHS ruling.

'We got you home, didn't we?' Andrea said. 'We were all living in his hospital room. I even got pregnant there,' she smiled.

'You got pregnant in hospital?' I said.

'Yes,' she said.

'Did you know that Sonny's condition was inherited?' I blurted.

'Yes. Both Talulah and Delilah were accidents.'

'But good ones,' I said. I was actually digesting the fact that Maff and Andrea had two more admittedly accidental pregnancies knowing there was an increased risk of having a second disabled child. What did that say?

The conversation moved on.

'Yes,' said Andrea. 'It was in hospital they said that Sonny is dysphasic or aphasic.'

'What do they mean?'

'Dysphasic means he is producing the language in his head but cannot communicate it, and aphasic means he is not producing the language in his head.'

'My money is on dysphasic,' I said.

'Roughly one year before the tracheostomy, they put in a stomach stent, so we can feed him directly into his tummy. It was taking him hours to eat a ham sandwich before.'

Up until Sonny was five and a half Andrea and Maff had fed Sonny themselves. But because his ability to chew and swallow were virtually non-existent he had become malnourished. Feeding Sonny took all day. Andrea would end up in tears, exhausted, just trying to keep her child alive. The paediatrician proscribed a nasal drip feed.

But getting enough calories through the nasal feed soon became an issue again. He needed the drip for fourteen hours a day, and he kept getting croup. The problem was, or rather one of the many problems was, Sonny's inability to have a productive cough. Not only did phlegm accumulate in his lungs, so did vomit, as well as food from the nasal feeding. His epiglottis was on the blink.

So on the advice of the paediatrician Sonny was given a gastrostomy. This meant that food was injected directly into his stomach.

'Now he has cheese and onion crisps blended up with milk and put straight into his stomach. He loves them.' Andrea's eyes shone with mischief as she kissed Sonny again. I suspected that blending cheese and onion crisps was not medically advised. Even before she had told me about her run-in with the NHS ethics committee, I had detected a certain delight she got from giving the authorities the run-around. Keeping the entire family, as well as conceiving a new member, in the hospital for eleven months, proved that. It was one of the many unusual ways in which she got to love Sonny. 'Nobody supported us,' she said triumphantly, and proudly. 'They all stayed in their safe zones.'

'So what changed that led you to escaping hospital?' I asked.

'What changed was the consultant,' Andrea said. 'We had lots of meetings, for months. But the consultant wasn't listening to what Sonny wanted. Then one day we were in the board room with the consultant, the physio, the lead worker and Frances who was liaison, and I got more and more insistent : You want listen to Sonny. You have to listen to Sonny. I was at the end of my tether.'

'But Sonny can't talk,' I said.

'That's what he said,' Andrea said. 'But the consultant just wasn't looking at Sonny, or listening to him. At one point I was going to kill him if he touched my son. But over the months he turned it round and started doing what we said. In the end he even kind of apologised.'

Maff came in from work, took off his coat and murmured something in Sonny's ear.

'We were right and we could look after him at home,' Andrea continued. 'Now we're friends with the consultant. He just didn't believe in us and Sonny. Did they, Mr T?' She gave Sonny a nudge. 'He treated Sonny like he was a case study. We just said Sonny's not your normal child. Not even your normal disabled child. I told the consultant, if you stop looking at all your charts and machines and blood tests and start listening to Sonny, he is going to lead the way. I said he wants to go home. All we need to do is leave here and go home. We need to get him home.'

'But they kept us there,' said Maff.

I could easily imagine how the hospital officials dismissed Andrea. She was just a mum who wouldn't face the truth about her severely disabled son. I'm sure they pitied her before finding her annoying and then probably scary. And at some point, when she would not budge from her view, probably around day 280 of the 307, they started doubting themselves. And then they realised that maybe Andrea was talking sense and that Sonny was, somehow, leading them.

'It must have been amazing when they relented and actually allowed you to take Sonny home,' I said. With impressive humility, both of them looked down and murmured that it had been. There was no smugness. It had been a harrowing year in that hospital. They had lived surrounded by sickness and death.

'Before we left they actually started to ask us for advice about other patients. Maff even did a lecture,' she added proudly.

'Who to?' I asked.

'The consultants, the doctors and nurses.'

'That's impressive,' I said.

'It was a nightmare,' Maff said. 'I couldn't get any words out. Everybody was sitting down in front of me, and there I was, dying in front of all the saviours,' he laughed.

'So what did you tell them in your talk?' I asked.

Andrea took over. It had surprised me that it was Maff who had given the lecture, because it was Andrea who was going to tell me about it.

'He just said we were patient and careful and never gave up, but also never pushed Sonny. It was Sonny that led us all. Didn't you?'

'We actually paved the way for ventilated kids to come out of hospital all over the UK who were being held there unnecessarily,' Maff said. 'They just had to train and to trust the parents. Not difficult,' Andrea said.

Sonny had stabilised and improved with the tracheostomy. His lungs didn't work on their own, but they still had their basic function. They got the oxygen into his blood and kept him alive. But the hospital would not let him go back to Frome without a care package, and the County Council were slow and unhelpful.

'We tried to stop getting institutionalised, all of us,' Andrea said. 'We couldn't just sit there day after day on that ward, so we took him outside, into the glass courtyard where people went to smoke.'

'We made it across the road,' Maff smiled.

'And we took him to the aquarium, against all of the advice,' said Andrea. 'We just decided to push it. To prove that we can do it. Give him a normal nice life. We are never going back into PICU again,' Andrea said quietly, under her breath. Later I realised that this was a very significant statement. It wasn't about how horrible hospital life had been, but about how there was a bar beneath which Sonny would not live. PICU was that bar. It was the only time I ever heard her say anything like that.

After 307 days in a hostel and hospital, home felt strange.

'The first night when he came home from the hospital ...' Andrea started, and broke off, remembering it, 'there was a bunch of strangers in the house.'

'Who were they?' I asked.

'The care team,' Andrea and Maff said together.

## 10

## Formula

The family were never again to be alone, and fully private, in their own home. The care team, it turned out, did not work for Andrea and Maff, or even for Sonny, but for the council, for the authorities: Social Services and the NHS. And the rules they enforced did not have to be agreed by Maff or Andrea.

I never heard Andrea complain about the rotating team of care workers who arrived in the house, but I quickly learnt that there were things you did not say and did not do when they were present. There was a faint impression that everyone was, if not under suspicion, then under surveillance. Each shift submitted case notes, which were reports on Sonny and any activities in the house which they thought might be significant, to the powers that be, who would then talk to Maff and Andrea about them if necessary. This was an additional burden on the many others the family shouldered.

'What were the areas of conflict between you and the NHS?' I asked.

'They told us to feed him dehydrated formula because it never causes blockages in the pipe, which they said blended food would,' Andrea said. I had dropped in for dinner and was sitting beside Sonny. 'That was nonsense. The doctors justified feeding Sonny chemicals by saying it was too costly to change the button when something went wrong.' The button was the thing attached to Sonny's tummy that you clipped the syringe tube onto. 'Maff just experimented with the kind of food we eat at home, and it's worked brilliantly. They had Sonny on thirteen meds when he left hospital. Didn't they? Yes! As well as making us feed him Nutricia. Nutricia stinks and made him vomit. It's what they give dementia patients. All manufactured. I thought there's no way I'm putting that in his body.' I bet she did. The combination of an organic, natural option and defying authority would have been irresistible. 'A lot of children who are fed Baclofen have to have an anti-emetic. But it was the food they told us to give him that was making him projectile vomit. At the time we were uneducated,' she laughed.

'What do they think of your blended feeding?' I asked.

Andrea waved her hand in the air dismissively.

The sweet and scented smell of another well-cooked vegetable curry was filling the house. Andrea called the girls to table while Maff poured the curry and some other vegetables into the blender and set it whirring. He brought through the results in a large bowl which he dipped a big syringe into. He drew back the plunger, filling it, then attached it to the tube.

'Where is it going into in Sonny?' I asked.

'It used to go into the stomach, but because of vomiting on the processed hospital food, it was moved into something called a jejunum bypass to enter his digestive tract.' I watched Maff push the plunger home. 'But when we got him home and gave him a blended diet we could move it back to the stomach.'

'He likes curry,' he said.

'It smells delicious,' I said.

'Does he ever have any food in his mouth?' I asked.

'No. He can't swallow. That could be dangerous.'

Sonny lived in a world without taste. He had the sense of smell, Andrea insisted, but he never tasted anything. The thought saddened me, though as I got to know the family better I always found it amazing that Andrea particularly would go out of her way to give him culinary treats, which he couldn't taste. To me, now firmly an inhabitant of Andrea's Narnia, it made total sense. You treated Sonny as you would want to be treated if you found yourself suddenly incapacitated like him.

While out on an errand, Andrea and I once stopped to get a beverage and she bought Sonny a hot chocolate to take home to him. She lifted the lid off his cup and said, 'That's not enough sprinkles,' returned to the counter and insisted on extra sprinkles. I looked at her in the queue waiting to be served while her coffee went cold and thought *That, Guy, that is madness or that is love*.

You assumed the best, you believed that his soul and his mind and his heart were no different to your own, and that if he couldn't taste the treats he could definitely appreciate them. And thus it was fun to give him these kind treats. Making Sonny sentient enriched our lives.

Supper at the house was always followed by clearing away, washing up, and then the click of the front door as two carers let themselves in, walked past us into Sonny's room, and settled down amongst the blinking lights for the night shift, sitting in the wing back armchairs, getting up to massage his lungs and suctioning out the fluids every half an hour until they departed at 7am. In the event of a carer's absence, Maff or Andrea did the night shift.

## 11

### Room of Broken Things

That summer, I went on holiday to a villa in Italy with some friends.

The Thompsons didn't go on holiday.

'Can you ever get away as a family?' I asked.

'Once we did,' Andrea said. 'To a carer respite centre holiday complex. We were all in one room. It was a Christian centre, but they were lovely. I'd like to do that again. There was a hospice which said it could look after Sonny if we wanted to go off on a holiday to the beach or somewhere with the girls and Finn, but,' she shook her head, 'the staff were very narrow-minded and scared of getting it wrong.'

'What do you mean?' I asked.

'They make the wrong calls and choices. We did it once and went to Wales, but after two days the hospice had panicked, called the hospital and they were suddenly giving Sonny antibiotics, which he didn't need if the suction was done properly. We were taught to do it by Bristol, but the nurses were too scared. They preferred drugs, and we had to pack up the holiday and drive back fast to stop them overcooking everything. Another time Maff had to drive back from Cornwall to rescue him. So, we can't really leave him safely with anyone.'

The way Andrea described it, she and Maff were protecting Sonny from an ever-present threat by faceless people who wanted to grab Sonny, place him in a bland and joyless council care home, pump him full of antibiotics and artificial powdered food, and then ignore him. It was Andrea's job to prevent this. And I was on her team.

At the villa on my holiday we were seven pink English people on the side of a desiccated hill. It smelled of thyme and sounded of crickets. My room had a thin mattress and nylon sheets, but the food and conversation were good. One wine-sodden hot afternoon, when the others were all taking a siesta, I explored the house and found the Room of Broken Things. Nearly all old rental villas have a Room of Broken Things somewhere, often down by the pool house, but if not there, in a small dark room in the house.

I found a low door by the staircase and pushed it open against a Z bed and two broken chairs. One had three legs, the other a broken back. There was a small high window blurred in cobweb. The bulb on the wall was broken so I sat on the arm of an old Squint sofa in the cool gloom beside two bedside lamps with broken necks. They had taken a pounding. A standard lamp was irreparably drunk. In front of me was a coffee table without its glass, a stoved-in waste-paper bin, a loo seat cover, three stained cushions and a royally ripped curtain. I guess the owners had abandoned plans to get them fixed but couldn't bring themselves to throw them out. The menders. The place where my mum took broken things. There were menders in my youth, but they didn't really exist anymore, at least not in the UK. These things would never be repaired or removed. I breathed in the scent of old pillows and deep and damp foundations.

Broken things always had a story. I imagined the shenanigans which accounted for this lot in front of me. The drunkenness, the sex, the tantrums, the spilt drinks, the dropped trays and shattered glass, and afterwards the undignified spat over the deposit involving petty lies with the distant and angry owner.

Upstairs the marble sitting room with the low pale pristine sofas, matching lamps, clean rugs and glass topped table told a duller tale. The guests had been striking poses and photographing themselves and each other, an event unlikely in the room below. Over dinner my friends asked me what I was working on and, as I told them about Sonny, I felt myself welling up. I didn't apologise but let them see as the fist in my chest began to open and something long and tightly gripped fell free.

I told them about the Room of Broken Things I had discovered. 'Sonny is the king of the rooms of broken things,' I said. 'His throne is his wheelchair. His story is more interesting than stories of unbroken things and people. And he can't be fixed and he can't be thrown away.'

## 12

## **A flash of colour**

I said to Zoe, 'Does Sonny have favourite TV programmes?'

'You love *Top Gear*, don't you?'

'Sure do,' said Sonny somehow. But he did say it. I got it.

'Do you like Jeremy Clarkson's jokes?'

An anxious look.

'Do you like the cars or the noise?' Zoe asked.

Nothing.

'Why are you not talking?' Zoe said. That was the kind of remark that after months in the household I took pride in not commenting on. 'D'you need a suction?' She pressed on his chest with that frightening force, and then jumped into action, changing pipes and flicking on the pump, finishing with a sweep of his mouth with the little curved pipe. 'Just give you some water, shall I?' she attached a big syringe full of water to another pipe under the blanket and pressed the plunger home.

Andrea came back in and asked Sonny what he wanted to do, but now she was signing with her hand as she spoke.

'What's that?' I asked.

'I sign as back-up. I use it more when we're out.'

I thought about this, because up till then there had been no suggestion that Sonny was deaf, or had any hearing problems. If she could make herself understood with sign language, it suggested that maybe it was words he had trouble with. I definitely thought he grasped meaning but could only get at it through a thicket of confusing and irrelevant stimuli. Like trying to catch a whisper in a blizzard. It often seemed as though it took about thirty seconds for thoughts to reach his face. We were on the other side of the thicket, trying to find a way through. Sign language was one of those attempts.

'He wants to watch TV. Don't you?'

'Does Mummy restrict screen time?' I joked.

Andrea looked at me as if I were insane, because I had used such complex language. 'Ask it in another way Guy,' she said.

I could see I had reached the outer limits of what was possible to ask, so changed tack. 'It would be good to do an activity with you,' I said to Sonny. 'What does he like to get up to?' I asked Andrea. I am, by now, acutely aware of talking about Sonny in the third person in his presence. The Radio 4 disability programme, which was really my first short glimpse into their world, was called, using heavy irony, *Does He Take Sugar?* But with Sonny there really was no other way for me to get solid answers, though I continued to try.

## A flash of colour

'Do you like swimming?' I asked. 'I like to swim.'

'That would be good. He loves swimming, though it's difficult with the tracheostomy, we're not supposed to take him in the water. The water can go down the tube into his lungs.'

'The carers don't approve?' I asked.

'Yes, it is against the rules. But we do it. Don't we, you rebel!'

It was the type of thing that some carers might submit a report about, but Zoe was sound. I could tell by how relaxed Andrea was around her.

'But we can go swimming,' Andrea brightened. 'We'll make it work. Won't we Sonny?'

Andrea went back to the kitchen, leaving me alone with Sonny. He seemed alert.

'I think swimming is a good idea. And I would like you to come over to my house at some point. Meet some friends.' He was watching me and signalling with those eyebrows and eyes. I couldn't be sure, of course, but it looked like he was happy with that idea. But as usual we were dealing with that almost impenetrable hedge between us. I couldn't quite see him. Occasionally I glimpsed him. A flash of colour between the branches. Then the undergrowth closed around him, or I moved and lost my sight line.

I looked at the boy. No, I corrected myself. Young man. He was shortly to be fifteen. He was a young man.

I said, 'One of the good things about going to the swimming pool is we can scope out some women, and you can get a good eyeful of some scantily-clad girls your own age. Wearing nothing but bikinis and smiles.'

And the moment I said that I saw Sonny through a gap in the underwood, in a clear gap between the trunks, through a break in the bracken and brambles. I saw him in a clearing, standing up, looking straight at me. A shaft of sunlight fell on the carpet of pine needles he stood on.

'Okay,' I said.

He was engaging with me, and he was saying, 'That thing you said about looking at the girls in their bikinis, let's do that.'

I laughed. Then I thought, shit I'm going to have to do it. I am going to have to go into the outside world with Sonny and receive all those looks which I gave the people like Sonny whenever I saw them and their carers - encouraging, polite or neutral as I tried to hide my pain, sympathy, fear and disgust. I was going to be on the receiving end this time.

By this point I would have told anyone that Sonny was trying to communicate in a meaningful way. He was giving signals, but he was doing it with a dodgy transmission system. It was as if I wanted to type *I can see you over there* and I typed the correct keys but this came out on my screen: *th see ov you*. Sonny was conversing in extreme Yoda, with only his face. When he tried to say *yes,* the word *nes* appeared on his features. When he tried to say *hello everyone,* he actually said, *gnnup ttel*. But after the time I had spent with him I was absolutely convinced that he was trying to converse sensibly and logically.

Zoe reappeared and said 'William has been taken up the Tor. The rugby team did it, and William's quite a weight.'

The Glastonbury Tor is a stone tower on top of a steep hill which resembles a small volcano. Forty minutes from Frome, it is a magnet for mystics, misfits, and the curious. There is always an ant trail of tourists ascending and descending it, and a bunch of people on the top tired and exhilarated from the thirty-minute climb.

'Who's William?'

'William is a friend from school. William has an older brother. Also at school.'

'They are both at the school?' I said.

'Yes,' Zoe said.

I swallowed. 'Well, we could do the Tor, it's always lovely to look out at the world from the top. But the swimming pool is my favourite.' I said that, hoping to cheer up Sonny.

Andrea went out into the garden to hang the washing. Family life went on around Sonny. Zoe and I focused back on him. The lad certainly kept you on your feet. I quite liked that. Zoe had produced Sonny's remote control car.

'I bought him this for his birthday,' she told me.

'When was that?' I asked, occasioning a classic Sonny scene.

Andrea had come back in and said to Sonny. 'You know your birthday.'

We all looked at him. I thought, right Sonny. She would never have said you knew your birthday without you being able to deliver. But I had forgotten Andrea's modus operandi, which was to plunge out of an upper floor window and believe she would land on the soft and giving mattress of love and optimism. Or even actually fly. She took Sonny, me and Zoe with her.

'Well, we know what day it is, it's the first, isn't it? Yes. Well done.'

We all exchanged triumphant smiles. So far so good. Yes, I knew what was happening but I understood why. We were riggers building our scaffolding to support the house as it was constructed. Sonny was the edifice, gently rising from its foundations, inside our support.

'What month?'

I leant forward, gathered up by Andrea's enthusiasm. A small part of me said, *we can't even be sure of yes or no, how is he going to use his eyebrows to say September?* I need not have worried.

'Is it January?' Andrea said, and managed to sound as if she didn't know.

I looked for cues from Zoe.

It wasn't January. I shook my head and joined in. 'No,' I said.

'Is it February?'

No, it wasn't February. My money was on March or April. It couldn't be November or December. No one had that much faith and love. How many years had this been going on? Nine? Probably longer.

'March?'

I looked into him. A wrinkling of the skin on his forehead. Anxiety. Not good. Worry. Was that a no, or a yes? Had we gone past the month? Surely not. Sonny now clearly looked up at the ceiling behind him. I had noticed him do this before and I had an idea it meant FORWARD or GO ON FURTHER.

Andrea went through the months one after another. When we got to September, a cheer went up from her and Zoe, and a smile seemed to flit across Sonny's cute face. I am not certain which one was first. A victory was declared. 'Well done,' I said. 'Brilliant.'

I thought about the man in the *The Diving Bell and the Butterfly*, the paralysed guy in hospital who is moaning about being cut off from the world when he can control his own eyes and eyelashes. One blink for A. Ten blinks for J. Twenty-six for Z. And he thought he had problems.

## 13

**Express joy**

'What're his stats like?' Andrea said.

She glanced at a digital readout on his ventilator. It monitored how much oxygen was in his blood. 97. Fine. If it went too low, they attached the pure oxygen from the tanks in the corner of his bedroom. Right now they were using air.

Zoe said, 'Let's play with your car.'

She set it on the floor and fiddled with the control pad on the tray attached to Sonny's chair. The car strained to move.

Zoe went and found new batteries. Then Sonny's hand was lifted and placed on the pad. The car set off across the shiny floor and crashed at low speed into the legs of the coffee table.

'Have you been drinking, Sonny?' I said, while I turned the car around so he could drive it back to his chair. It was hard to see if he was driving it. Zoe put his hand on the pad. Think of a sock full of sand. I know that's tough. But Sonny cannot move his fingers or raise his hand at the wrist or elbow. The question I was trying to answer was whether he had any control over that car.

## Express joy

He seemed to express joy. Pleasure in the car. There was only Zoe and me with him. Andrea was on the phone in the kitchen talking about arrangements for the kids. Zoe placed the limp hand on the pad and the car shot forward until it hit an obstacle, and then I turned it, and Zoe picked it up when it hit the chair.

'Yay,' I said as the car, a red and black Bugatti Chiron, trundled in first gear back over the wooden floor and hit the sofa.

I bent down, turned it round and stood up, smiling at Zoe.

I tried to see if Sonny could see the car. I wasn't certain of how well he could see. His eyes sometimes roamed the room as if he couldn't see properly. What does properly mean in this context? I don't know. Anyway, he was looking down at the floor in front of his chair and appeared to be watching his car and his face appeared to be smiling. And then I noticed something else. I stood up, and felt a strange but undeniable sense of joy filling the room and warming me, softening my heart. It was born from the simplicity and beauty of my friendship with Sonny.

Zoe went about her business. I said, 'You can leave me on my own with him.'

'Okay,' she left the room. I put the door to, but didn't close it.

Without the usual conversation and Andrea's laughter, the room fell quiet. Out of the silence bubbled the whirr of Sonny's ventilator, as reassuring as an aquarium pump. I started to stand up, but knew I was happy to stay in the quiet with him, so didn't leave his room. Unusual feelings of contentment, balance and gratitude washed through me. For some reason, he was a balm to my sores.

I realised I could tell Sonny anything. I guess I felt safe. I thought he was listening, but I didn't know how much he could understand. I was bored of talking about football, and tired of always checking in to see if he was catching my drift. I proceeded now on the basis that he could understand me, but was unable to express that. And I am sure it was as tiresome for him as it was for me, trying to work out what he was communicating and failing.

I said, 'I like being here with you. You calm me down.'

I left a gap, but didn't bother to try to put his reply into a multiple-choice questionnaire to see if I could get a reaction that satisfied me.

I don't know if he smiled. He was looking at me in the eyes, that was for certain, before his gaze roamed the room and across the ceiling again. I figured that most people simplified their thoughts before articulating them to him. If I were Sonny, and my theory about his cognitive ability was correct, that would madden me.

Andrea popped her head round the door.

'Everything all right?'

Express joy

She came in to rearrange the blanket round his feet. 'He loves having someone to chat to, don't you? Are you happy Guy's here? Yes.'

*Someone to chat to.* Fox, the frisky little terrier jumped up onto Sonny and turned in circles on his motionless legs and played with him as if he were perfectly healthy, as if Sonny was in the habit of taking her for a walk.

If you build it, Sonny will come. I am surprised Andrea didn't put shoes on his feet. She was constructing a reality, like writing a play, with everything in place but the main character. We were the actors on Sonny's stage, running through our lines, waiting for him to appear from the wing and join us. Until then, the technicians, co-stars, and bit part players like me continued our run through of the drama, as if Sonny, the star of the show, was present in the theatre.

I read while doing my research about a woman called Liza who had a son called Jamie even less responsive than Sonny, who took two weeks off work to read him *The Chronicles of Narnia*, 'just in case he could understand it'. I knew that Andrea read to Sonny. I didn't know if he could understand the story, but I could understand Andrea. She was putting everything in place for a sentient childhood, and whispering with her love and devotion, *Come on Sonny, it's here for you. We are waiting for you. When you're ready.*

Jamie's father said of his unresponsive son, 'It's raw just being a person without trying to impress or achieve or accomplish anything. It's pure being. In a totally unconscious way he is what human is.'

I felt exactly the same as I stood beside Sonny. It was a moment of pure being.

'You mind if I sit on the bed?' I asked.

'—'

I was still conditioned to feet moving to make some space, but they remained where they were. I settled myself right on the edge, so as not to press on them. His feet were small; they had never been used.

Andrea put her head around the door.

'You can leave us alone,' I said. 'I'll shout if we need anything.'

She left us alone. The ventilator sighed and wheezed. 'It must drive you mad the way she talks for you all the time, though you know she does it out of love. My mother talked for me all through my childhood,' I told him. 'She answered questions aimed at me, told people what I liked and didn't like and what I wanted to be when I grew up. She was just proud of me and loved me, like your mum. It was fucking annoying. And I could actually talk for myself. And leave the room. Luxuries you don't have. It must piss you off. It would piss me off. Mind you, you're mum's super-hot.'

The aquarium pump silence fell again. I could tell I had said something wrong.

I took a breath. 'Look, I can say your mum is attractive without breaking your family up, ok? I met her at a wild party. She was always on her own. I assumed she was single, but now I know why she was always on her own, because Maff was at home keeping an eye on you. She's not going to leave your dad, right? Or leave you. Or the family, because of people fancying her. It's only fancy, not love, not even adore. Just fancy. It's quite normal. Well, very, when you see her from behind picking a toy off the floor. Sorry, I momentarily forgot I was talking about your mum. But don't worry, nothing bad is going to happen. I assure you it's not reciprocated. You know what that means, don't you? Yeah. That. As soon as I met your dad and saw what a great guy he is, and how happy they are together, I no longer thought of her like that.'

I looked at him and his eyes flicked off me for an inspection of the door frame.

'But your dad's pretty hot too,' I said. 'Okay. That was just a joke to wind you up. But you were right to bring it up,' I said. 'Okay?' I gave his foot a little squeeze.

We communed a bit longer listening to his pipes gurgle.

'Women,' I said, wanting to get it off my chest, and realising there were few more reliable confessors to talk to than Sonny. 'They're the delight of my life. You like girls? Well, you're fifteen and you look to me like you have an eye for them. It's just a feeling. I bet you get a girlfriend. Don't be surprised I say that. What! Of course you will. If you want to.'

I let him process that nugget, and felt the atmosphere lighten as it soaked in.

'I had a friend in a wheelchair once. He was the only other man I ever knew who couldn't walk unaided. He was called Quentin Crewe. He was an excellent writer. Really good. And I tell you Sonny, the girls loved him. They flocked to him.

'It may surprise you, but you have many advantages over other men when it comes to the opposite sex, and don't you forget it. No. For a start you can't do the one thing women hate men doing: leave them. And you can't give them too much trouble. Plus, and I know this to be true, you're a fucking brilliant listener, on top of which, you have a beautiful face, lovely skin, and a very attractive presence. I'm not gay, but I can feel it. Well I'm not that gay, except when it comes to your dad. Okay! Okay! That was a joke. That is not going to happen. I absolutely promise you.'

I heard Andrea on the phone in the kitchen.

'I can tell you,' I said to Sonny, 'with absolute certainty, when the time comes, you'll get some action. You know, a bit of rumpy pumpy. Of course you will. If you want it. And don't you worry, sex is so subtle, and so divine, there are lots of different ways of doing it, and you will find a way that suits you with the right girl. My friend's nanny used to say, "for every pot, there's a lid", and believe me there's a girl out there who will be a lid to fit your pot. Don't be so surprised. Sex is nothing like what you may have seen on a screen. It's spiritual and creative and has no rules. You will discover that. Still, in the meantime, when we go swimming we can scope out some women in bikinis, eh?'

The door opened. Andrea popped her head around it and said 'What are you two talking about? Not football again? Honestly.'

I flashed Sonny a smile.

'We're just chatting,' I said.

Andrea stood there.

'A private conversation,' I added.

She tutted and left the room.

'You are a remarkable person, you know?' I told Sonny. 'You engender love. You encourage protection, and nurture kindness. You bring out a delicacy in me. Well, sometimes. And patience, neither of which are qualities I've been overendowed with. When I am with you, I quieten down and turn up all my senses to commune with you. I feel like a bird watcher. I like it.'

## 14

### Eye-Gaze

On the 7th May 2021 I received this text from Andrea:

*Sonny had an Eye-Gaze assessment today. Do you remember me telling you that I've been trying to get one for him for a few years and I believe it will allow him to communicate in more ways than I ever thought possible? Well I am so pleased to report that he totally smashed the initial assessment. He wowed the assessors! They are coming back for more communication play in a month or so. I am so very happy, Guy. This is what he needs to have a voice. I'm on a high! All is good xxxx love and more* ♥.

She attached a minute or two of footage of Sonny having his first test on the equipment.

The Eye-Gaze was a bit of computer hardware and software that made it possible to control a cursor on a screen with your eye. The screen had a voice function. In this way people could talk using only their eye. Stephen Hawking had one.

It was hard to see exactly what was going on in the clip, but there was – it being Andrea – an atmosphere of ebullience and triumph. I turned up the volume and played it again, expecting to hear the computer croak some words which emanated in some way from Sonny, but I couldn't hear properly. Andrea was on a high, though, so it had to have gone well. It went well enough for Sonny to earn himself a shot at getting an Eye-Gaze for himself. As far as I could tell, this machine would enable Sonny to talk, though it might take a bit of practice for him to learn it. That would be a seismic moment. His first words at fifteen. But Andrea had told me that the Eye-Gaze was an expensive piece of kit.

The reason Sonny was fifteen before he had a crack at getting his own machine was because the government were sparing about handing them out. You had to prove it wasn't wasted on you. I guess they had a limited number of machines, and they wanted to make sure they were not left unused in somebody's house. Sonny did have access to one at his school, but it was shared, and he never seemed to get on it. Why had there not been a campaign to get him one of his own?

I wondered about this as I drove towards Frome, through Somerset landscape coming into leaf and blossom on a glorious May morning, through the chic gentrified streets of cute Victorian houses which were admired mainly for the astonishing increase in their value, and out onto the newish estate where the Thompson house stood on the flank of a hill surrounded by other homes.

The dread I had felt driving to my first meetings with Sonny had been replaced after ten months by excitement at seeing him. It was an astonishing privilege to be present when Sonny said his first real words. For on this early summer morning he was being given the final Eye-Gaze computer test.

I got there early. Sonny was in his room being showered, so I stood in the kitchen talking to Maff about my life, and noticed how quickly I started talking so intimately with him. In this house the façade was thin.

Then it was time to see Sonny, in a green t-shirt, red neckerchief, black trousers and smart black and red socks. Sonny's socks were always clean. Of course. His hair was amassed in curls on his head.

'He's got a quiff going on,' Zoe said.

'All right?' said Andrea, 'Christopher Reeve?'

Sonny seemed happy and positive, but how could I actually tell? It still mystified me. The feeling in the room was definitely positive, and I was happy to be there. Zoe pushed him through to the lounge and spun him into position. 'It's like we're having a dance,' she said.

In the lounge two women were unpacking computers and plugging in cables.

'What's happening?' I asked Maff.

'I'm not sure,' he said.

I sat on the arm of one of the two leather family sofas, as worn and welcoming as the family they served, and got out my notebook. I wrote *What are Sonny's first words going to be?*

I was a late talker. I made do with one word, *Onga,* until after my third birthday. It covered everything, and I seem to remember I was perfectly happy with it. But I was sent to speech therapists who wanted me to say *cat*. We didn't even have a cat. It was not a word I had need of. Onga was.

Later in my childhood I was often told about Lord Curzon, the creator of the British Empire in India, and who was still in the 1960s much admired, who also didn't talk until very late. He was considered retarded as a child and treated as a baby. He was allowed to sit with the grown-ups because he never said anything. One night he burned his mouth on a spoon of hot soup and the woman next to him made a great fuss of him, consoling him like an infant. *Are you all right diddums?* The four-year-old Curzon stared hard at her and produced his first ever words: *Thank you, madam, the agony has now abated.*

What were Sonny's first words going be?

It was exciting. Fifteen years of trying to make himself understood was coming to an end this very morning and I was to be there to witness it.

What would he say?

Then I thought, Oh no. What if his first words were *Guy fancies mum*! Or, worse, *Guy fancies dad, he told me.*

The Eye-Gaze lady was ready. She was a large bustling woman not over endowed with empathy. The screen was wheeled in front of Sonny. He looked stressed. Not surprising really. I approached him and whispered in his ear 'Don't throw me under the bus, Sonny. When I said that stuff about Andrea and Maff it was on the strict understanding that you would never be able to talk.'

The Eye-Gaze lady looked at Sonny and said, 'That's a nice smile,' and went back to her computer.

Andrea saw me whisper to Sonny, and assuming they were words of encouragement gave me a grateful nod. Then she closed the curtains while I sat back down. With the room dark except for the screen there was an element of entertainment about proceedings.

'At the last assessment there was a real progression,' said the Eye-Gaze lady. 'He asked for toast and fried eggs. This kid's amazing. Do you remember? Liverpool, Great! Man U. Bad! Yes. That was excellent response. The team said let's bring him up! How's his hearing?' she asked.

'Pretty good,' Andrea said.

'Sight?'

'He's referred to vision support. He hasn't seen anyone for some time.'

I didn't know any of that. Typically, Andrea hadn't told me. It allowed negativity into Sonny's life.

'He wears glasses because he's short-sighted,' she said. 'Sometimes it's a bit of a guessing game,' she continued. I thought: no kidding. 'I don't know if it's suction, needing something moved behind him, or nappy. I have to go through everything,' she smiled, heroically, I thought. A smile that after fifteen years of trying to read her child, only Andrea could produce. It was a smile that would not have looked out of place with the remark *sometimes he puts his shoes on the wrong foot*. 'He really wants to say he wants to go to the toilet.' Yes – we were at a heart-breaking level of communication. I avoided Andrea's eyes because these were delicate matters and none of this had been said so explicitly.

'How about literacy?' the Eye-Gaze lady asked.

You're ticking boxes, love, I didn't say. But it was a cruel question to ask. We were trying for *can I go to the loo, Mum,* not 700 pages of *The Order of the Phoenix*.

'It's not something we've really explored,' said Maff diplomatically.

Then Andrea said, 'We read captions on films out to him,' making it out like that in some way this was an achievement for Sonny. I thought *You absolute beaut, Andrea.*

The Eye-Gaze lady looked up from her computer. 'Any activities of interest that can motivate?'

It was quite a painful question, if you had the most passing knowledge of Sonny. Activities weren't really his gig. He couldn't actually move. This didn't stop anyone in the room of course.

'Sonny really likes music,' Maff said.

The Eye-Gaze lady nodded and smiled.

'He likes music,' agreed Andrea, and put in an extra mile for Sonny. 'He likes to listen, and play.'

'Animals and dinosaurs.'

'What else do you like?' the lady said.

Maff said, 'Fish.'

'Oh – I've got too many things in the box now Sonny.'

Andrea said, 'He really likes bees.'

I thought, *did she say that just to muck up the woman's boxes?* I did think I had sensed an element of a stand-off between the two parties since the Eye-Gaze team's arrival.

'Okay....' The Eye-Gaze lady looked up. 'Medication?'

'He's not on any medication,' Andrea said. Adding with a hint of triumph, 'not since *2016*.'

'Because we feed him real food,' Maff said.

The Eye-Gaze lady, batting for the opposite team, let that ball go straight through to the keeper.

Andrea said 'Sonny? Water?'

'He's had it,' said Zoe from the corner.

'What are you looking for?' I asked the Eye-Gaze woman.

'The Special Needs Team issue a device and offer goals if criteria are met.'

'What are they?' I asked.

'Well, it's an NHS funded device. So, it's up to them. But I think he'll pass. It just has to be intentional.'

So there it was. The bar had been set. Come on, Sonny, I thought, you can do it. You just had to avoid being random. Come on my son!

Andrea's chin was resting on Sonny's head so she could see what he was seeing.

The room fell quiet, and the system was activated by Sharon, the Eye-Gaze boss, and Rachel her timid assistant. I could see the screen from behind Sonny. They moved it into his eyeline, wherever that was. With Sonny you were never quite sure.

'This is the fiddly bit,' the Eye-Gaze lady said.

To Zoe, Andrea said, 'Just put it in the bag and have it in the bag all the time.' I didn't know what she was talking about but understood it to be another example of how alert Andrea was at all times around Sonny. Keeping the team up to the mark. She sat down in an armchair, leant back and crossed her legs underneath her.

'It's exciting,' she said.

The Eye-Gaze woman said, 'Maybe we need a bit more volume.' I supposed because we had not heard the computer and therefore Sonny, say anything.

I spotted the extra-large cursor before it shot off the screen and didn't reappear. Then it moved back near the edge of the screen, on which there were a few icons. Then it stubbornly remained motionless. The Eye-Gaze Lady tapped her keyboard.

'We are still going at point six of a second?'

'I will make it slower, otherwise you get those mishits.'

'Last time he got into a flow. I was crying with excitement,' Andrea said.

Nothing happened for quite a long time. The Eye-Gaze lady said, 'That's frustrating.' To Sonny she said, 'I can see you looking at them. What are we on? Point six. Put it down to point five.'

I took the opportunity to get round in front of Sonny, so I could see him. He looked to me to be focused on the screen. Like he had intention.

His eyes moved around and the cursor must have moved because the computer croaked some words:

'Awesome,' it said, in Hawkingese. 'Great.'

I think Sonny smiled.

Then the machine said ... no, then *Sonny* said:

'Special, special, special. Great. Awesome.'

## Eye-Gaze

And then he went quiet again. I didn't know quite what to make of it. To be honest, I wasn't convinced. I knew Sonny pretty well, and I had him down as a more reflective guy. For me, there had to be a more thorough examination of the equipment, leading to proof that it actually worked before he would be feeling so effusive. Or maybe I had it wrong. He was as upbeat and gung-ho as his mum. Sonny was like Andrea! I'd never thought that.

They put onto the screen the football card, with icons of players and supporters.

Eye-Gaze lady said, 'Over here are your sounds,' and moved the cursor onto an icon.

'Come on England,' intoned the machine.

The cursor zig-zagged until the Sonny machine said:

'Goal. Goal. Goal. Come on England. Red card. That was a dive.'

'Can you find the clear button?'

Sonny cleared the screen.

I said, 'Well done.'

Then silence.

'He's overwhelmed with options,' the lady said. 'We're going to slow it down a bit.'

Another card came up, with animals on it.

'Look at a bird,' the lady said.

I went through the kitchen to come round and see Sonny from the front again. In front of the sink, a boy with a hoody was pouring milk into a bowl of cereal. This was Finn, Sonny's seventeen-year-old brother. I had not met him before, but had felt his presence mainly from his footfalls on the ceiling. He hadn't come down to say hello to me, the way Talulah and Delilah had. He had made it quite obvious that he was not that excited about my project. That made sense to me. From Finn's point of view Sonny, however much he loved him, must have been somewhat of an interruption to life. And here he was again, hogging the attention. I didn't have time to stop and exchange pleasantries, so introduced myself and quickly nipped round the corner.

Sonny was checking out the ceiling, cool as he could be, but there was a whiff of failure.

'Do you want to try it one more time?' the lady said. 'Pop that balloon.'

Oh how we all yearned to hear that pop. But none was forthcoming.

'I think we need a recalibration.'

When it was set up again Sonny said 'Special.' Then 'Special.' Then 'Special' again. We all sat in silence listening to him. In a way it was a fairly logical thing for him to say, if he was actually saying it. He had no doubt heard himself referred to as special all his life. And, particularly as I attributed a strong sense of irony to my friend, a rather clever and definitely funny thing to say. But on its own, repeated over and over again, it challenged that interpretation.

I watched Zoe's face as the word rang out from the box. Her belief and devotion were also unwavering. That was love. A professional love, but special, as Sonny would say.

We went off football and animals and on to music. Icons of instruments populated the screen.

The shake of a tambourine raised morale. Then the bird came back on the screen, the one Sonny hadn't clicked on before.

'Sharon!' the machine said.

'Sorry, that was me,' Sharon said in the darkness.

Maff and Andrea went to make a cup of coffee. I figured they were used to things going slowly. I went through to say hello. They did not look downcast. I wanted there to be a narrative arc like a firework. I thought Eye-Gaze was going to ignite a rocket, but the blue touch paper fizzled and went quiet.

Next door Rachel said, 'It's not working again. I don't think it's you.'

The machine said 'I like drum. It is really loud.' I put my head round the corner.

Sharon said, 'That was me.'

People were still talking for Sonny, but I heard what I thought was a happy gurgling from him. You never knew, maybe he had wanted to say he liked a loud drum. But the heady days of *Liverpool, great! And Man U Bad*! were a long way behind us.

'It looks like he's looking,' Sharon said.

But nothing emerged from the machine. She fiddled for a bit. I was thinking, this is a bit of a shitshow. The kit's rubbish.

Then the tambourine rang out.

'We're back in the room,' I said.

Bang bang bang bang went the tambourine. If he'd actually been banging it that loud someone would probably have said 'Sonny, please,' but we revelled in the din. It sounded like Sonny. I think all who knew him thought that.

Then he brought in the drum. Boom boom boom. Then the rattle of the tambourine.

Then the machine said, 'LISTEN.'

Andrea said, with a quaver on her voice, 'did he just say listen?'

Sharon said, 'No. That was me.'

Then the machine, or Sonny, said 'Stop. Stop. Stop. Stop. Want. Stop. Stop.'

After a shocked silence Maff softly said, with such kindness in his voice, 'the Eye-Gaze altogether?'

Words then gushed out:

'Want. Want. Want. Wash. Brush. Brush.' My mind was haring off in every direction.

'Stop. Want. Stop. Want. Stop. Stop.'

Well, that was pretty clear, I thought, but bloody disappointing.

'Wash. Brush.'

Andrea said 'Wash the brush. You want me to wash the brush.'

Maff said 'He can't mean that.'

I was thinking that talking Sonny may be more difficult to deal with than silent Sonny. I hadn't thought of that. But I was not convinced Sonny was talking, not at least in the sense that Andrea, Maff or I were talking. If he was it must have been annoying that the first thing he said was disregarded.

But Sonny was off. He was either accidentally or by volition pulling more icons onto the screen. 'Want. Brush. Help. Hot. Stop. Wash. Water. Cold. More. Dirty. Dry. Towel.'

I wondered if in the sheer thrill of finding his voice he was just enjoying saying random words. We were all trying to make sense of them, and none of us referred to his repeated STOPS.

Then he said, 'HELP. HELP. HELP. HELP.' That many times, because I was making notes and each time he said it my writing was getting more ragged as I felt pain and sadness, and my hand grew heavy like meat. 'WANT. STOP. STOP. STOP. WANT. STOP.'

I wanted it to stop too. If it were any other child you'd jump up and say what's wrong? But none of us did. I think we all felt we knew Sonny wouldn't actually be saying he wanted to stop what was such an amazing opportunity for him and us. And if amongst his first words were HELP HELP HELP HELP it was just too ghastly to contemplate, at least right then. Poor Sonny. Oh my Sonny. Calling for help, in the ruins of the collapsed building. With the ceiling pressed against his face.

But Sonny wasn't finished. 'Radiator,' he said. I looked round for the radiator. It was mainly hidden by a table. There was nothing remarkable about it, to me. 'Radiator,' he repeated. 'RADIATOR. RADIATOR. RADIATOR. PEACH.'

That made me sit up.

'RADIATOR PEACH. RADIATOR PEACH. PEAR PLUM PLUM PEAR. PEAR. STRAWBERRY. PEACH. PEAR.'

There were about twenty icons on the screen. Andrea got up and pointed to some. 'What about down here. What do you like? Banana?'

'Radiator. Peach.'

Then the cursor went to the off button and clicked it. Sharon turned it back on.

'Peach. WANT WANT WANT WANT.'

I figured that want would be the most powerful word for someone in Sonny's position, denied it for all of his life. It made sense that he was enjoying saying it. It was his way of saying this is me. I have my own wants. Want. It made sense to me.

'He keeps turning it off,' Sharon said, turning it back on.

I said nothing. It was quite complicated enough without me weighing in.

Sharon was proceeding on the basis that Sonny was not expressing his true thoughts.

I said nothing.

All through this seismic hour, Sonny of course had remained totally still.

Sharon said, 'I have to go now.'

Sonny said, 'GOOD.' We all laughed nervously.

As they were packing up I asked Sharon how she thought it had gone.

'If we can get some goals on it, I think he can make progress,' she said. 'You can see from his facial expressions his understanding of language.'

I thought that there may be a conflict between her goals and Sonny's wishes.

I said nothing.

Maff came closer for a suction. He moved quietly and gently and carried it out with heart-breaking tenderness, compressing Sonny's lungs, feeding the pipe down his windpipe and bending forward to activate the pump.

'Are you a bit tired?' he asked, and answered, 'No?'

Sharon presented a bit of paper to be signed. 'This is consent for the video. We use it for training purposes.'

After the Eye-Gaze team had left, in a tacit admission that the session had not gone as well as we all hoped, Andrea said 'If it's not NHS we'll go down the charity route.'

Andrea and Maff never minded letting people help them, but I sensed they were resistant to accepting cash from donors. Sonny's extension at the back of the house which included a bedroom, bathroom and hoists to move him around, cost £54,000 to build. He was getting too heavy to carry upstairs so it had to be built. They received a disability grant of £30,000 but that left them £24,000 short.

'We crowdfunded it,' Andrea told me. 'Maff didn't want to do it, he said it felt like begging,' she added.

'I didn't,' he said.

'You did,' Andrea said.

'I don't remember saying that,' he said.

'The council said we'll give you 20k if you can raise the rest of the money.'

'Well Sonny will get an Eye-Gaze free on the NHS. What he has done is on the back of only two sessions,' Sharon said as she packed up.

'How much does it cost?' I asked.

'The camera is a thousand. The table is between four and five. The software another thousand … it's about eight with the mounting.'

Sonny was crying. Andrea dabbed away his tears.

'It's three to six months till his next assessment,' she said.

## 15

### Relationship history

Andrea and Maff invited me over for dinner later that month. I was grateful that they were being so co-operative, friendly and creative with the project. I hadn't shown them any of what I had written and they hadn't asked to see it.

Sometimes I felt uneasy about what they would think. But I knew I was in good faith. It was only later when doubts began to gather on the horizon that I started to worry about the consequences of what I had started. Then I would wonder if the clouds were darkening or dissolving.

Talulah and Delilah rushed me at the door. They had a lot to tell me. Delilah, the youngest one, six years old, looking out cannily from under a cascade of tangly brown hair, sat upside down on a chair describing everyone in her class to me, while Talulah watched me cautiously, I expect working out if I could be trusted.

They had been to Young Carers and they wanted to explain all about that. It was a support group for children who look after a disabled sibling or parent. Then Delilah told me about a school outing they had been on, and how Mr Hime her teacher had pretended he had locked them in the bus and lost the keys.

# Relationship history

I passed Finn in the kitchen buttering toast in the air. He had a bathrobe with a hoody on, like a boxer.

'All right?'

'Yuh.'

I'd heard Maff and Andrea beefing about Finn not getting a job or getting off his arse but, by the standards of my family when they were his age, he was pretty dynamic. Up and out of bed by 4pm? I would have taken that as a win.

I went on through to Sonny's room, the girls chattering in my wake.

It was growing dark outside and the lights were low around the bed. I had been told that Sonny had had a cold, and it had been a difficult week for him. Andrea had lost a few nights' sleep looking after him.

'Radiator peach,' I greeted him. 'Heard you've had a tough week,' I said. 'Been on the oxygen, right?'

Andrea had explained that during his cold his ability to absorb oxygen through his lungs had become so impaired they had had to put him on a tank of the stuff, basically to keep him alive. I could see a number flashing on a digital readout. It said 97. If it dropped too low they had to mix in some pure oxygen from white cylinders in the corner under Virgil Van Dijk.

'I'm sorry about that,' I said. Fox galloped into the room and leapt via the chair up onto the bed, partially to defend Sonny, partially to get a good look at me. She was allowed free rein with Sonny and padded all over him in his chair and bed, with nobody stopping her. She ran with a hop and a jump into the lounge when the girls tried to tie a scarf around her neck. When the room was empty, I tipped the door shut with my foot and sat down on the end of the bed. I took a glug of my wine. I was pleased to be alone with Sonny to tell him my news, to amuse and, hopefully, outrage him. I understood that everyone wanted to talk about football and cars to him, because it made them feel safe to be on topics that were encouraged by Andrea and Maff. His whole room said you can talk about football and cars. I am sure Sonny liked those subjects, but they presented such a limited world to him.

So many of the adventures most fifteen-year-olds were having with illicit, or at least naughty, activities, whether it was copping off with a girl, dabbling in soft drugs, lighting a fire in a deserted building, or necking a bottle of cider, were off limits to Sonny. I wanted to show him that the world was not bland and beige.

I decided to dive straight in with women problems. 'I'll give you a bit of background here, my friend,' I said. 'I warn you, my relationship history is not pretty. I don't know why. You may be a settler, a family man, like Maff and Andrea, but it wouldn't surprise me if you were actually a bit of a player. I don't know what it is, I have a feel for spotting them, I suppose it's because I'm a bit of a legend myself, though I wouldn't use that word to anyone but you. Nothing wrong with having an eye for the ladies, I hasten to add, nothing at all. We get a bad rap, guys like you and me. Ladies' man – you've got it written all over you.' I gave his foot a friendly tap. 'A little bit of flirting lights up this gloomy world we are forced by birth to inhabit. Makes the ladies glow and the gentlemen go. Don't ever let anyone tell you different.'

I raised my glass to him.

'To you,' I said. 'And all flirts.'

Then I drained it.

I gave him a quick update on my relationship history. He seemed interested enough and for me it was great to talk. To talk and be listened to was actually a bit of relief as, emotionally speaking, my life had been a tangle of brambles recently. And although I had used counsellors in the past it was much better not to be faced by some dowdy divorcee in a classic *1970s* armchair who was half interested and half annoyed by me but charging me *120* quid all the same. Sonny was a much better therapist. He was the king of the questioning silence. And totally free.

Twenty minutes later I was just saying, 'So, well, the answer to my problem was obvious really, though it took weeks to work it out. But it was right for me, Sonny: I had to shag them both, it was my only option.'

Andrea popped her head round the door. 'Everything okay? Call me if he needs a suction.'

'How will I know?'

'He gets distressed and goes red, through lack of oxygen.'

'I'm colour blind,' I say.

'You'll know.'

She closed the door. The aquarium pump wheezed. I checked the read out.

'Ninety-eight,' I told Sonny. 'You're looking good.'

There was a comfortable silence.

I thought about what I was going to talk about next and tried to think of something I wanted to get off my chest but couldn't mention to anyone else.

'Did I tell you, or did you hear, that I've been nominated for a book prize?' I looked at him. 'It's called the Everyman Bollinger Wodehouse Prize for Comic Fiction. I've been wanting to win it for years. It is incredible really that I have finally got on the shortlist. I pretend it doesn't mean much to me, but it does. Pathetic, aren't I? My publisher said you can forget winning it, Guy, have you seen the other people on the shortlist? They are all basically young, hot and brown, and there is at least one Muslim there, so you haven't got a hope. Old, white, middle-class and English? They're not going to give it to you. You're not saying what the brand wants. I'm never gonna win it, Sonny, no matter how good my book is.'

I paused, gazing at Sonny, and was struck by a thought.

'I would be a shoo-in if I looked like you Sonny. Though you're not black. You've got that against you. It is my luck to be writing at an unfortunate time for old white blokes. It was actually shit when the white men were in charge and only old white men got prizes. I'm not saying bring back those days. They were even shitter really... basically no one black or brown got a look in, and quite a few talentless old buffers did quite well just because they were white and went to the right school.'

I stared at him. 'Did you just snigger?' I said. 'Are you calling me a talentless old buffer who just went to the right school?'

I hadn't actually sensed him sniggering, but I was operating on the *if you build it, they will come* scheme of discourse, creating the space for Sonny to inch in to.

I squeezed his motionless ankle. 'You cheeky fucker,' I said. 'Hey, but you could be right. You could be. What say you, we go into partnership? We sit here chatting away as we do, right, and I write a book, and I announce to the world that you wrote it by dictating it to me. You will be the writer.' I paused as what I said sank into me surrounded by a cloud of bubbles. Then I croaked: 'It will be your photograph on the shortlist.'

I gazed in wonder at the lad. Pipe in the neck, eyes a bit wonky, cute smile, oxygen tank against the wall. How in this new glorious era could Sonny ever be refused a literary prize?

This meant a total rethink of the entire project.

'We will walk the awards season, Sonny. Or roll them. What do you think?'

You're not going to win that prize. Getting on that short list is the nearest you'll get.

'Yeah,' I said. 'I'm not going to win. I thought you'd agree. Thanks for telling me nicely.'

The door opened and Maff came in holding a bowl of something delicious.

'Everything okay?' he said.

'Yeah, great,' I say.

'What have you been chatting about?' he said.

'This and that. What's that?'

'Dinner.'

Maff pulled the blended stew up into the syringe and fitted the end to a transparent tube that disappeared under the blanket.

He said, 'Can I show the button to Guy, Sonny?'

I said, 'No, I don't think that was an enthusiastic yes from him. And I totally understand why. We don't know each other well enough for me to see that. I'm fine not seeing it.'

I said that for two reasons: because I wanted to err on the side of respect in my new friendship, that I wouldn't want my dad pulling up a blanket to show some bloke my tummy valve, and because I thought that was what he had said. How, I don't know. Silently.

Maff pushed the plunger home and the food shot down the pipe and into Sonny. Soon it would appear in his nappy. It seemed brutally mechanical, when other parts of the boy were so mystical and inexplicable.

We started to talk about the football season. I had not abandoned my ambition to get to the front row of a football match to see Liverpool play, and I had had had my eyes on the European Cup Final in Istanbul. I was already mentally writing heart-rending letters to anyone I knew or knew of who had a private jet and asking them if they could lend it to me to give the poor lad the excitement of a live game of football for once in his restricted life. I then thought, why stop at a private jet and googled the best hotel in Istanbul and made a note to write to them asking for a complimentary suite for myself (and a room for Sonny) as an act of humanitarian philanthropy. Sonny was turning out to be the key to rather a lot of activities which I had previously thought out of my reach. I was even thinking of getting the whole trip sponsored by Bollinger. It was the kind of set-up the big brands would be gagging for.

But a problem arose. Liverpool's season had fallen apart.

Getting Sonny to the Stadium in Turkey looked a lot easier than getting Liverpool there. When we got knocked out in the quarter finals by Manchester City the gig was up for *2021*, so I rescheduled for *2022*, though we still had to finish in the top four places of the Premier League table to qualify for that competition. This would normally be a formality, but *2021* had been such a calamitous year for the club that at one point we were struggling in eighth position.

After twenty-seven games it was looking like no European football for the Reds after a campaign undermined by injuries and a catastrophic run of home form including successive Anfield League defeats. But in April the boys had started winning, and both Chelsea and United had started to stutter.

Maff gave Sonny a second helping. I watched the plunger and thought about someone squeezing that much liquidised vegetable stew into my intestine at that speed and immediately wanted to go to the lavatory. It hurt me to watch it, but Maff knew what he was doing, and Sonny seemed fine.

'Does Sonny ever get anything in his mouth for taste?' I asked.

Andrea was standing at the door. 'Sometimes I put a bit of sugar on my finger, or lemon. He likes that, don't you Sonny? But he has no swallow reflex, so we have to be careful. That's why we have to use the suction tube, to clear the saliva from his mouth.'

Maff pushed the plunger home. The room was now full of the scents of good and wholesome food.

'Halfway through the season we were washed up,' I said. 'And then like the champions we are, we came back, and we may even end up in the top four.'

'Incredible,' agreed Maff. 'Sonny and I have watched every match. We remember that loss at Burnley, don't we Sonny?'

I thought, if Sonny could talk what would he say? He'd say: *My dad watches every single Liverpool game with me.* And I was glad the room was growing dark, because I started tearing up at that thought. I guess it was the double devotion: to each other and to Liverpool Football Club. The double loyalty. You'll never walk alone. That was the Liverpool Football Club motto. A touch infelicitous when you thought of Sonny's condition, but the point still stood: we look after each other, we Liverpool fans.

'It's looking like we might make the Champions League after all next season,' said Maff.

'Do you remember the West Bromwich Albion game, Sonny?' I asked.

How could I ever forget it? he said. In the final minute of the match our keeper had run the length of the pitch and scored the winning goal with a header.

After the match, I had stayed glued to the TV, watching Jürgen Klopp, our charismatic manager, give his verdict on the night. 'It's big. If someone told me five, six, eight weeks ago we can finish the season in third - it was out of reach, barely possible.' I knew Sonny would adore Klopp. 'Fighting through this and finishing here in third is the best lesson you could learn in life,' said Jürgen. 'From nowhere to the Champions League in five weeks is a massive achievement.' Jürgen would understand and appreciate Sonny, without question. I added a meet and greet with Klopp to our pre-match schedule. Of course Jürgen would want to talk to Sonny. Who could refuse? And meet Sonny's interesting carer: me. That would put the cherry on our evening's entertainment. I checked to see where the 2022 final was being held. Krestovsky Stadium in Saint Petersburg, Russia, on 28th May. Interesting location. I had not been to St Petersburg, but I knew there was a magnificent hotel there, in the old style. Andrea could come with us. No. Maff would come. He did the football.

We left Sonny to sleep beside the graphs and numbers which grew brighter in the dark.

While Maff, Andrea and I ate the same stew, the front door buzzed.

Andrea called, 'Come in Charlotte,' and two women walked through the house, past us into Sonny's room and closed the door.

'Is that off duty for you two now?' I asked.

'Yes. Ten o'clock. Until seven in the morning when we take over again.'

## 16

### I couldn't explain how

I went away to write up my notes. I told friends what I was up to. They all asked me if Sonny was sentient, and if he could make himself understood. I said he was, but I couldn't explain how.

I drove over to Frome on a late summer morning. While I had been away in the tropics on a five-week writing and boozing trip, the hawthorn had faded and the hedges and woods had grown into their full English summerness. I was met at the door by The Young Carers.

Delilah said, 'I'm going to marry my bed.'

I said 'Good choice. Cut out the middleman.'

Talulah, who was nine, was in the middle of schoolwork. Delilah arranged herself upside down in the chair to read a book. Sonny was busy in his room, having a massage. There was something about him that reminded me of an entitled aristocrat from the sixteenth or seventeenth century. Or was he like one of those boy Chinese Emperors who ruled over 500 million people but couldn't tie their own shoelaces?

While we waited for him, his sisters showed me the books they liked.

'This is called *Rainbow Grey*. It's a book about a teenager, with one purple and one blue eye. I got given it by a charity called Purple Elephant.'

I had noticed how many charities played a part in the Thompsons' lives. The scepticism I had developed over the years about charities, basically around a suspicion that they were only in it for themselves, was softened when I saw how useful and kind they were in this household.

'Don't tell me,' I said, 'the boy with the funny eyes gets bullied, and then someone sees how beautiful he is in his difference.'

Talulah stared at me, her mouth open. Then she said, 'No. That doesn't happen.'

'Right, what other books are there here?' I said, hoping Andrea had not heard me.

'This one is *The Boy, the Mole, the Fox and the Horse*. It's got lots of nice messages,' said Talulah. She looked at a page. "When the dark clouds come, keep going," she read. "It's hard to be kind to other people, but being kind to yourself can start now."'

'Do you believe that?' I asked.

'Of course,' she said. 'Listen to this. The mole says, "I have learnt how to be in the present." "How?" asks the boy. "I close my eyes and focus." "What do you focus on?" "Cake," said the mole.'

'I like that,' I said.

'Mr Hime is leaving school.' Mr Hime was only ever spoken about with total adoration. I knew from the way she spoke of him that he was a brilliant teacher and lovely man.

'I'm sorry,' I said.

Andrea was singing a song in her husky voice in the kitchen. She appeared in the lounge looking gorgeous, smiling from ear to ear, radiating her usual joy.

'We've had trouble with a carer. Charlotte has gone.'

'Does that mean you have to do nights and extra shifts?' I said.

'Oh yes,' she smiled. 'Of course.'

'I'm just amazed how positive you are,' I said.

Talulah looked up from her book and gazed at her mum.

Andrea said. 'I think you've just got to make the decision to be a miserable fucker or not and that's really ... what's the point? I don't see the point in wallowing in something you've just got to deal with.'

Talulah smiled and went back to her book. I thought, this family is so tight, and so resolute and so full of love. You could almost sunbathe in it.

We started talking about Sonny's swimming trip. I was brought down to earth by practicalities.

'I'm not so keen on Charlton Farm,' I said. It was an institution set up for people like Sonny, a kind of all-inclusive resort for people with SMD. It was fully equipped and fully staffed. Sonny went there from time to time to get some days away from the family and give his mum and dad a break from looking after him.

'When Sonny is at Charlton Farm, that's when we do the things we can do without the wheelchair,' Delilah told me. There were quite a few activities in this category because Sonny's chair weighed twenty-five stone before he sat in it.

'Is there a public pool in Frome?' I asked.

'Yes. But Frome don't have a hoist,' Andrea explained. 'Unless he can be lifted in. But then it's getting him out, he's quite heavy. We did ask for a hoist, but it never materialised. Some of the pools are a bit twitchy about Sonny swimming. They put loads of cones around him, and everyone avoids him,' she said, without a hint of pity. Or anger.

I thought, I wouldn't mind seeing that. To face my own fear and shame, and I guess to see others'.

Andrea went to give a hand to Sonny. Through the gap in the door I glimpsed him being hoisted towards his shower. I watched Talulah reading with her lips moving.

'Delilah. Can you get me some saline please?' Andrea said from next door, and Delilah slipped off her chair to get it.

'How would you describe your life, as Sonny's sister?' I asked Talulah.

'Our life isn't hard, it's just different. Some people have got it worse off.' When she was an infant and toddler Talulah used to sleep with Sonny. You can see that now, years later, from their almost eerie sense of communication with each other.

Delilah said 'Okay, what do you need to know?'

'I don't know,' I said.

Talulah put her book down. 'His favourite colours are red, orange and yellow.'

'How do you know that?' I said.

'He tells us,' they said together, without hesitation.

'How does he tell you?' I said.

Talulah said 'So ... we'll say is it red? Orange?' and her hands started signing as she spoke.

'Does he understand sign language?' I said.

She ignored that question. Which was odd because Andrea brushed me aside when I asked her about her signing. It was a secret, magical, inexplicable communication aid. 'He'll frown at the ones he doesn't like and smile at the ones he does like,' I was told.

'And to you that's quite clear?' I asked

'Yeah, yeah,' they both said.

'He loves Weetabix,' said Talulah with absolute certainty. He doesn't even eat.

Delilah said 'His favourite carers are Zoe and Nuala. He thinks it's really funny cos he says to Nuala, "You're sacked".'

'Does he?' I said.

'Yes,' they both giggled.

'How do you know that?' I asked.

'People ask that quite a lot,' said Maff from the kitchen. I was touched at the way both Maff and Andrea kept an ear out during my talks with the girls, but never answered for them or interfered in our conversations.

'Yeah,' said Talulah.

'We sometimes ask if he wants to sack Nuala. Sonny always says he wants to sack Nuala,' said Delilah.

'Always with a big smile,' said Maff, now standing at the door.

'He seems pretty happy,' I said. 'Does he seem happy to you?' I asked Talulah.

'Not being able to do normal stuff you'd think he'd be sad but he's really happy. We do loads of stuff with him and that makes him really happy.'

'What a nice sister he's got,' I said. 'Two nice sisters.'

'Three,' said Talulah. 'Including Fox. When we have friends round they just sort of stare at him. They're always a bit scared.

My friend Sophie talks to him like I do. With Deli's friends we have to say, "don't worry he's not scary just a bit different but just like you" and they don't really understand that.'

'That's what I'm trying to understand and to explain,' I said.

'I know,' said Talulah. 'What else? Sometimes I'll suction his mouth. I can shake him and suction his mouth but not in his lungs, you have to be fourteen for that, but I will. I'm going to be ten in a week's time. I can do his bagging and help turn him. When I was very, very little I'd always sleep with him. This might sound a bit silly but I help him watch TV. When he has options on interactive TV he tells us what he wants to do.' Deli nods her head as her older sister talks.

'You are both very good at giving him his voice,' Maff says.

I suddenly felt overwhelmed by what was before me. The harmony, the love, the kindness and compassion brought tears to my eyes, which I didn't want any of them to see so I fumbled for my hanky. Tears of joy and pain. I, too, wanted Sonny to have his own voice. I wanted him heard.

'He does cry a lot, too,' Talulah said.

'Why, do you think?' I asked.

'Sometimes he cries because he really needs a suction and he can't breathe properly,' she said. Then she changed the mood. By this time she was totally in charge of our interview. 'We go to this club called Young Carers. With people who have a sibling or a parent or grandparent with a disability and you go there to take a break. I have looked after Sonny loads, and when he doesn't have a carer, I'm his carer. And I'm reading a very encouraging book, because it helps you believe in yourself.'

'What are some of the best things about having Sonny in the family?'

'Mum's teaching me to do physio on Sonny, and many children won't be able to experience that. Like, we were already loads ahead of people by knowing this stuff. I go to pick up Sonny from school and I see all his friends and they are normal to me. If I wasn't his sister, I wouldn't think that. I would be quite scared of them. So that's good. And if I've had a bad day I go and hug him and I sort of like tell him what has happened. I know he can't do anything but he sort of comforts me in a way that no one else can see it. You need to have sadness to know what happiness is.'

The masseur emerged from the bedroom. I introduced myself. She was called Lorn. She looked a strong, confident, middle-aged no-nonsense woman.

'I'm writing a book about Sonny.'

'What kind of book?' she asked.

'I want to explain him to the world, I guess,' I said. 'Would you have five minutes to talk to me?'

'Yes,' she smiled, sitting on the arm of the family sofa.

'How long have you been massaging Sonny?' I asked.

'It must be nearly two years now,' she said.

'What mobility does he have?' I asked.

'Sonny can move one of his fingers on his left hand. When I do a muscle strip on the side of his arm his finger twitches and his face lights up. I always get a smile response.'

'Wow,' I said. 'You get right through.'

'Oh yes – you just got to look at his eyes,' she said. 'Plus, when I do a skull release I can feel it all the way down the spine, and he beams.'

'How is he doing that?' I asked.

'We are communicating with far more than our physical body and its movement and our speech. We have a whole energetic body as well.' I nodded enthusiastically. Here was the explanation I had been after. 'Whether or not you are into all that you will pick stuff up, especially if you are quite open to it.'

'Before meeting Sonny I used to be sceptical about it,' I said. 'But he's changing me.'

She paused and then said, 'It's probably why you're doing this. It's probably why this is happening for you. That's your challenge. The universe has gone "there you go, try this".'

I swallowed. 'Do you think so?'

She smiled knowingly and nodded. Then she started packing the bag at her feet. 'Oh yes,' she chuckled. 'Oh yes.'

I said, 'I've got this awful feeling that Sonny's going to start teaching me a lot of new stuff about life.'

She stood up, put out her hand. 'Good luck,' she said as she shook mine.

Sonny emerged from his room on his chariot, auburn hair flowing, his cheeks glowing after his session with his personal masseuse.

We chatted for a while.

What does that mean?

I told him about my conversation with his sisters and spoke about our swimming plan. I told him I wasn't so keen to go to Charlton Farm because it seemed too clinical.

'But I am keen to do the football match. But let's start with a home game, at Anfield. Let's pick a group game in the Champions' League. When the groups are announced and the draw is made, we will choose a good match. How about Liverpool-Barcelona, at Anfield of course, with you and me within talking distance of Lionel Messi? Listening to Mohammed Salah call out to Mané for the ball.'

A thought crossed my mind. I leant closer so nobody but Sonny could hear. 'Now, will you tell Maff that, and you choose the match? I won't say anything to him, so it's down to you.'

It was a test. I wanted to see if Sonny was capable of communicating to Maff that we were all going to a UEFA Champions League match at Anfield.

'You tell Maff and I will organise the rest.'

## 17

## **Brutal environment**

I had only ever been with Sonny in his home, either in his bedroom with him lying down before sleep, or in the lounge, where his chair took up a lot of the space. For over a year, I had been getting to know him in his comfort zone, building trust. Or at least that's what I told myself. In fact it was my comfort zone we were staying in, and I knew what I was scared of: going outside, and particularly being seen, with Sonny.

My first time out in public with him turned out to be a severe testing in a brutal environment. I went with Andrea to Talulah and Delilah's sports day. Sonny was coming straight from school with Maff to join us there.

As we drove in her Mini through the prosperous streets of old Frome, Andrea surprised me by saying she didn't like doing social events with parents and teachers. Maybe it was because her girls didn't attend the local primary school but a smart little private school at the leafier end of Frome. It was a lovely late summer afternoon, with white puffy clouds in a blue sky, a bright sun and a warm breeze.

'How come the girls are at a fee-paying school? Are your parents paying?'

'Delilah and Talulah are on full bursaries,' she said, raising her eyebrows and smiling. I wondered if that was anything to do with Sonny, but said nothing in case it seemed uncharitable to the girls.

We pulled up at a cricket pavilion on an immaculate green sports field, edged with mature oaks and a white picket fence. Parents had spread rugs and were opening picnic boxes. The shadows of the poplars beside the pavilion were long. Children ran up to bowl in the nets. I looked at the very English summer scene. Despite being mid-September it was a hot day. The men were in shirtsleeves, the women in summer frocks. It was actually a picture-perfect scene of English middle-class life, and in the faces of the adults sitting on the rugs I definitely noticed the smug ambition that private school parents sometimes fail to hide. I walked in with Andrea. She was wearing her usual brightly coloured and slightly out of fashion leggings and a t-shirt, which that day had some cooking stains on it. She knew surprisingly few people.

'Come on,' I said, 'they're serving booze.' I shepherded Andrea toward the bar.

The headmistress finished her little talk about toilets, safeguarding, and health and safety, and was standing by the table with the flutes of wine on it.

The headmistress gave Andrea a look that said, 'Oh it's you.'

In the queue we got chatting to a new parent, a blow-in from London, whose child had only been at school a fortnight. This was Caroline, who wore a hat, lipstick and shoes with block heels. I noticed that she was on her own and in possession of a picnic rug, picnic hamper, and friendly manner. Andrea and I were soon sitting on her rug eating her prosciutto and drinking her bubbly. Sonny had not yet turned up, and the girls darted up to us from time to time. Caroline had previously lived in Hackney, a fashionable part of London for hipsters. She airily told us that her husband had bought a landmark building in Frome town centre to develop into studios and flats. She attached herself happily to Andrea, me and the girls, and while she told us how wonderful her life was, I felt a mixture of anxiety and excitement about the thought that Sonny was about to turn up.

Andrea looked at her phone and said, 'Maff's here.'

'I'll go and give them a hand,' I said, getting up and walking between the dappled picnickers. As I went through the gate in the picket fence I saw Maff's black van cruising down the road looking for a place to stop. I caught up with it beyond a bus stop. The door was open and Sonny was on the tail lift, Maff holding the controls. Sonny was in a red neckerchief and cap.

I wanted to do something practical, a sure sign I was feeling anxious, so I looked for a drop kerb. I had scoffed at dropped kerbs for all my life but now, with Sonny in the motorised chariot, I blessed one when I saw it. We crossed the road. I swallowed and smiled as we approached the idyllic scene ahead.

I scanned the crowd as we went through the wicket gate in the palings. I realised that I must have looked like Sonny's grandpa to strangers. It was a painful spike at my vanity, ego and identity. I wasn't an outsider, with a professional duty to be alongside Sonny. I was in the family. It was, yes, my DNA in that wheelchair. That would be in the background of the minds of everyone who saw me.

This was what I was expecting: people glancing up, then looking away and murmuring something before carrying on with their picnics. An old man who shook his head slowly from side to side. A toddler who pointed and shouted out, 'What's wrong with him, Mummy?' I had been scared to be out with Sonny, scared to see him humiliated, misunderstood, ignored or even abused. His vulnerability made me protective.

I didn't want to run away, or try in any way to detach myself from Sonny (for instance by walking ten feet behind and writing some bullshit in my notebook.) I stayed absolutely at his side, trying to remain calm and relaxed. But not a single adult nor a single child stared open-mouthed at us. The wheelchair handled the going admirably, and although Sonny rocked from side to side there wasn't going to be the ghastly spill I had imagined when I first realised we were going to have to negotiate uneven surfaces. It had been a dry autumn and the ground suited Sonny's mount.

I waved as we drew closer. Caroline's Waitrose picnic lay opened. Her pink mules were placed neatly by the tassels of the rug. I stood firmly by Sonny's side, wondering what I was going to feel and do in this unfamiliar moment. It was a tough first gig: a private school function, featuring hundreds of perfect children with picture-book families. I could have done with breaking myself in with a trip to the stained shopping centre in the middle of Frome where I could count on at least a couple of fatties in mobility scooters to take some of the heat off me and Sonny.

I knew how Sonny would be: the same. He was always the same. With all those people not looking at him, but surely noticing him, he remained the same. That was one of Sonny's superpowers: his ability to be Sonny in any situation. Had I been wheeled, as a fifteen-year-old boy, in front of a smart primary school on sports day, with the pupils all jumping, running, shouting and laughing, I would have been very unhappy. I would have been sorry for myself. Sorry that I couldn't scamper about and make friends and throw a ball or kick a ball or jump a hurdle. I would have been angry and bitter and upset. But I looked at him and there he was, my buddha in a neckerchief: implacable, solid, unperturbed, and proud.

Talulah dashed up, shouted 'Hi Sonny,' pressed her cheek against the back of his hand, murmured something and ran off to play. I was watching Caroline first register Sonny, then confirm, as Andrea kissed him, that Andrea was his mother. Maff, Andrea and I stood proud and solid beside him.

Caroline saw all this and was not alarmed. Hackney was the metropolitan borough of Woke Central. Thank goodness. Plus, she was on a mission to make friends and be liked. This was a chance for her to show what a tolerant, cool woman she was. It was a chance for all of us. We joined the picnic as welcome, but not particularly special, guests. The general public had passed the test.

I suspect that there were many parents on the picnic rugs silently giving thanks for not having Sonny sitting by their rug, in their family. They were thinking what a parent of a SMD boy I read about said: "Sometimes I think, god! That's for life; all the way out to the horizon there's nothing. He is not going to get married, have kids, become a grandfather, buy a house. He's going to do nothing a person does which gives life texture."

I stuffed another one of Caroline's Waitrose cheese sticks in my mouth. Sonny had led me to a state of kindness and openness, and given my life texture.

And we were about to try and create an edifice in the landscape of Sonny's own life: a football stadium. A big one. Called Anfield.

## 18

## You'll never walk alone

It was in October that I applied to Liverpool Football Club for tickets for Sonny and his two carers – Maff and me. Maff was a serious footballing man. He had played the game at a good amateur level and coached the youth team at Frome Football Club until Sonny's demands made that impossible. Maff and Sonny watched every minute of every Liverpool game on the TV on the arm above Sonny's bed.

Andrea said to me: 'I could say the house is burning down and Maff wouldn't move during a football match.'

I drove with the printout of an email on the passenger seat beside me through the drying autumn woods, along the bristly fields, down into the valley of Frome and the house on the hill. As I waited for Sonny to emerge through the double doors, sitting on the edge of the sofa holding my piece of paper, I got a feeling of being admitted into the royal presence.

'Listen to this Sonny,' I said. 'Dear Bella Ainsworth' - she's the disability officer at Anfield - 'I write to you on behalf of my friend Sonny Thompson, who, although fifteen, is unable to write himself.'

'My name is Guy Kennaway. I am a writer of books, and I am currently engaged on a project involving Sonny who has a condition sometimes called SMD, which stands for Severe Multiple Disabilities. Sonny has been a Liverpool supporter all his life. It gives him a lot of strength. He watches every game dressed in strip and draped in the scarf. Although Sonny has limited communication, particularly verbally, he is a truly committed fan and follows the ups and down of the Club closely. I attach a photo that gives the idea of Sonny and his devotion to the Reds.'

This was a photo of Sonny on match day wreathed in his scarf, wearing the Standard Chartered home strip of *2020*, with another strip folded on his bed. I was standing behind him beside Sonny's 'This is Anfield Liverpool Football Club' badge poster, with its prancing liver bird with a sprig of something in its beak. Sonny looked excited and focused. His main ventilator and a battered oxygen tank were in sight on the floor, and his air pipe clearly visible. I was confident it would work its magic on Bella Ainsworth and the tickets.

'My book is an attempt to portray Sonny and describe his life. My idea is that by bringing him into the mind of the reader, people will be more understanding of Sonny in particular and disability in general. I really want to end my book on a high note, and I know there are very few things Sonny would enjoy more than to see a Liverpool game at Anfield.

'I do not know how much of the actual game Sonny will be able to take in because his vision is not perfect. But if we can get tickets close enough to the pitch, I am sure he will see some of what is going on, and I KNOW for a fact that he will feel the Anfield family warmth, and will benefit from that huge and moving rendition of You'll Never Walk Again, all of which I am sure he will never forget—'

Andrea, who was cooking with Delilah, shouted through, 'Not you'll never walk again! You'll never walk alone! Alone! Not again.'

I glanced back at the paper in my hand. I had actually typed *You'll Never Walk Again*. Shit.

'Oh yes,' I said, blushing. I hoped Sonny hadn't heard but of course he had. The club anthem was sung, clearly intelligibly, by the mass of supporters before every home game. It was probably the only song Sonny was certain of the lyrics. 'I don't know how that happened,' I said to Sonny in his wheelchair.

I looked back at the paper.

'Sonny and I are asking if we can buy tickets and have provision made for Sonny's physical challenges. We are not that picky about which match we see, but it must be a home match because foreign travel is absolutely out the question until I write to Raheem and beg a ride for Sonny on his private jet (I assume he has one).

'Let me know if there is any other information you need to advance our case, or whether we should be addressing our request to another person. With very best wishes, Guy Kennaway and Sonny Thompson.'

I looked up at Sonny winsomely.

Maff said, 'And Raheem Sterling doesn't play for us anymore. But apart from that it's good. It's good.'

I felt sweat appear on my face. Sterling had left the club years ago. He had been at City for at least two seasons. It was beginning to look like I was a fake Liverpool supporter. Maff looked at me, and I wondered if he was thinking, *Did Guy say he supported the Reds just to get in with Sonny and me, and do his horrible work?*

With my phone in my hand I googled Liverpool's upcoming fixtures and said to Sonny, 'After Christmas, I mean I think we should wait for the new year before doing this, we have these home games: Brentford on the fifteenth of Jan ...'

Maff said to Sonny 'Ooh. Are you interested in seeing Brentford?'

We looked at the oracle. There was some facial movement. Months later I realised that this was a telling moment, but at the time I brushed it off as a typical Sonny conversation.

As usual it could have gone either way, but I was aware that both Maff and I did not want him to choose Brentford, a side of little pedigree. We didn't want to slog with Sonny in the van all the way up the M6 to Anfield to have the trip wasted on seeing the lads thrash a bunch of semi-professional upstarts like Brentford.

Maff said, 'Not Brentford?'

I said, 'Wait till you hear the other options,' and didn't look up in case he had the expression he used for being unhappy, like when he was in dire need of suction. His expression of distress.

I said 'Eighth of February, Sonny, listen to this. Leicester! That'll be a good match. At Anfield, obviously. Eight o'clock kick off. Under the flood lights.'

'He's usually asleep by the end of 8 o'clock kick offs,' Maff said.

'And it would be nearly eleven by the time we got back to the hotel,' I said, 'though the floodlights are magical. But I guess in January it's going to be dark by the end of afternoon kick off anyway so we will see them.'

'So, Brentford it is, right,' said Maff. 'What else?'

'Saturday nineteenth of Feb: Norwich,' I said. We had railroaded Sonny over the Brentford match, although I never confirmed this with Maff. And we didn't really offer Norwich to Sonny either, because a bit like Brentford, neither Maff nor I wanted to see any minnows. We wanted big fish. Although Maff and I were talking in front of Sonny, we had stopped checking in with him. That sounds harsh. But football is football.

'Maff,' I said, 'West Ham on the fifth of March, and, wait for it, Man U on the nineteenth. Both afternoon kick offs.'

Maff and I smiled at each other and turned to Sonny. 'Now those sound like good fixtures,' we said. 'Don't you think? Yes? Yes?'

'Yes!' I said, looking at Sonny. 'That is a definite yes.'

'Let's try for them. Man U would be amazing but I doubt there's seats available ... even for Sonny,' Maff said.

It was agreed that that was what I would do. Agreed, that is, by Maff and me.

As I drove home through the dark, deserted streets and out between the spooky hedgerows of the country lanes, I detected an uneasy feeling about what had happened with Sonny. I thought in some small way I had been dishonest with him, and myself.

Sonny had not expressed a preference to see West Ham or Manchester United. I just said he had. And that niggled.

You could say the whole scheme of dragging Sonny to a match so I could enjoy it was dishonest, but it was predicated on the idea that Sony himself would love it too, so I think excusable. But I had not detected any enthusiasm from my friend. I buried my doubts.

## 19

## **A woman at an old wooden desk**

A month passed and I didn't hear back from Bella Ainsworth at Liverpool Football Club, so I re-sent the email with a short covering letter. This time I received a reply:

*\*\*This is an automated email\*\**

*Thanks for contacting Liverpool Football Club. We have received your email and will look into it as soon as possible. We have created a case reference in the Disability Ticketing Department and put it in the subject of this email, which you should include whenever you contact us about this enquiry.*

*Kind regards. Fan Services. Liverpool Football Club.*

I tried calling but was told to email. I felt ignored and sidelined. I had thought the photo would do the trick. I was wrong. When Andrea and Maff asked me how the Anfield trip was coming along, I said, 'We seem to have hit a bit of a brick wall,' and they didn't look surprised. It was a brick wall they were familiar with and had been looking up at ever since Sonny was born.

I wrote a tougher letter to LFC, in full finger-wagging patrician mode. I pointed out that this book was eventually going to be published and maybe even serialised, and that their casual treatment of Sonny, whose case for tickets was so strong, would not look good. Even as I pounded out the letters on the keyboard, I could not help feeling the powerlessness of Sonny's position. Let's be frank, nobody would care at all if Sonny didn't get tickets. He didn't have a voice, and mine was certainly not loud enough to make much difference, and in the final analysis people wanted to talk and think about other things.

The Disability Ticketing Department? Who were they kidding? Liverpool Football Club was a huge, heartless global business. I pictured their offices: rows of rooms with glass walls in which people had meetings about TV rights, image rights, million-pound sponsorship deals and VIP catered boxes costing ten grand a match. How would this so-called Disability Ticketing Department fit in there? It was probably a woman at an old wooden desk opposite the toilets whose main job was cleaning. I started editing my email, throwing in some insults about their treatment of the disabled fan.

Luckily, before I hit the send button on my ill-tempered rant, I received an email from the club.

*Dear Guy, Unfortunately all disabled tickets have been allocated for this season, but we are happy to confirm that Sonny will be allowed tickets for a match next season. The reason for the delay was that we had to accommodate two disabled supporters whose life expectancy was so short they were given precedence. I hope you understand. The cost of the three tickets will be £6.90 each, and they will be on the front row by the pitch.*

*In the meantime, can you please supply:*

Confirmation from the Department for Works and Pensions of your entitlement to the middle/higher rate of either mobility or component of care of Disability Living Allowance. If you now receive the Personal Independent Payment (PIP) you must be on the enhanced rate.

A letter from your GP confirming the nature of your disability.

With the news that the tickets, which usually sold for a £150 each, were going to cost twenty quid for three, I was no longer in high dudgeon about Sonny's treatment, but was nevertheless in low to mid dudgeon about being asked to prove how disabled he was. Surely the photo said it all.

I forwarded the correspondence to Andrea who sent me back some harrowing paperwork about Sonny's condition from the Bristol Children's Hospital, and a brusque sentence saying he was too ill for a GP and dealt directly with the consultant at the hospital.

That should do, I thought, but curiosity made me pick up the phone and call the Disability Ticketing Department to ask why they needed the paperwork.

A very friendly young woman called Shelley, who knew about Sonny from the correspondence, laughed when I asked my question. 'I can see you are a bona fide case, but you would be surprised how many supporters we get who are not in good faith.'

'What do you mean?' I asked.

'We've had cases of fans putting their mate in a wheelchair and throwing a blanket over his knees to get these disabled tickets, so we have to just check, you see, to be certain.'

## 20

### The cot, the bedding, the rattles, the bottles

During term time, Sonny went to school near Bath, about half an hour from home. One day I went on the morning school run to see the place. It was a newly built, expensive looking building with bold steel curves, plate glass and varnished wood with the feel of a well-funded arts centre or theatre. Attached to it was a light and modern café where the senior pupils worked behind the counter or waiting at tables to get work experience. It was, like Sonny's diligent carers, a standing testimony to how far this country has come in its care of the disabled. I had never seen a school that looked so well maintained.

I was made to wait in the café, where I was served a cup of coffee by a careful and nervous trainee waitress, while Andrea and Maff checked it was okay for me to go into the school. Some other boys and girls were loading a metal trolley with sandwiches to sell at break. Andrea had shown me a photograph of Sonny accompanying the trolley on his work experience day.

It turned out, because of safeguarding and health and safety issues, the school would not let me in. Apparently, I needed a DBS to set foot inside. This acronym stood for Disclosure and

Barring Service and was designed to find out if somebody had a criminal record. I was turned away at the door while Andrea was having sharp words with a woman whose arms were folded in a way that made me think we weren't going to win this argument. I had never been viewed with such suspicion.

I approached the two of them, ignoring the woman's killer look. I did not understand the fears of the teachers and nurses.

'You have not been properly vetted,' she said.

'You mean you have not approved me?' I asked.

'Exactly,' I was told.

'But if you only have writers and artists that have been approved by the NHS looking at your work, how can you expect the public to believe them? I am independent, but I come in a spirit of positivity and openness. Surely a quick look around to see where Sonny has his classes will do no harm?'

I was turned out, and sat on a low curved brick wall while more futile argument went on inside. But the trip was by no means a failure. As I sat on the wall, a touching scene began to be played out right in front of me. Not the one in which Andrea behind the glass gave someone sitting at a computer hell, but the one where parents dropped their kids off at school.

Each child was at this school because they couldn't keep up at a regular school. When I saw the first van backing into the parking space, I expected to see someone like Sonny lowered on the ramp, but the door slid back and a girl of about twelve and a well-dressed corporate mum got out of the front. Mum embraced the girl and watched her walk safely through the school doors. Then more cars and vans arrived, each depositing a child, some in light wheelchairs they could propel themselves, some who were pushed up the drop kerb to the doors where they were met by teachers. Some limped, some looked down at the ground, one up in the air – most moved in an unusual way. The variety was extraordinary; much wider than at a conventional school.

Each parent bid goodbye to their child and returned to their vehicle to turn the key in the ignition and get on with their lives. From their appearance, the situation weighed more heavily on some than others. Remaining motionless on the wall, seeing all these parents, whose worlds I had glimpsed into, knowing Sonny, I felt successive waves of pain, love, sadness, despair and hope break on my heart.

These parents were not just the group who had disabled children. They were more than that. They were the parents who had disabled children and had stood by them.

A British couple who I read about in my research called Jason and Elinor (names changed) left their baby behind at hospital. At five months of age they noticed that, on top of epilepsy and a worrying lack of development, their daughter's eyes started flickering, and took her to a paediatric neurologist at the NHS for tests. The consultant said that it was likely that Beccy would never walk or talk. It was a consequence of getting blood poisoning in the womb. They ran some more tests on the child, including a CAT scan. The result of the CAT scan was that Beccy, in the words of the doctor 'strictly speaking had no intelligence.'

Elinor and Jason already had a daughter aged two, who was at home, hearty and healthy.

'I did a very heinous thing on the first night,' said Elinor. 'I said, "I'm not staying". As I walked past the other parents, I did not meet their eyes. I was hanging up my halo. I got in the car and drove home.'

She was advised by a lawyer that because the birth had been so negligently managed they could sue the NHS for at least £3 million, which would cover Beccy's care costs. 'But I hoped that Beccy would be allowed to die.'

That weekend she took Beccy from hospital, but just to get her baptised, then returned her. To Elinor, the doctors' relentless focus on life seemed almost sadistic. Elinor called a lawyer and checked if she would be at risk of losing her first child if she abandoned the second to the system. The answer was she wouldn't.

On the day Beccy was due to come home, Elinor did not go to the hospital to pick her up. 'I'm not the right mother for this child,' she told the hospital.

Elinor and Jason had returned to the hospital to explain to them that they would not be taking Beccy home. The doctor

## The cot, the bedding, the rattles, the bottles

asked if Elinor had ever had thoughts about harming the child. Elinor replied that she could not deny that she had. The staff were kind and understanding, the atmosphere gentle. Elinor said to the nurse, 'I do love her, you know.' The doctor said, 'Let us take the burden from you.'

As the parents drove out of the hospital, Elinor wanted to turn back but Jason said, 'It's her or me,' and they drove on, Elinor crying silently.

When they got home they threw away the cot, the bedding, the rattles, the bottles, the baby clothes, the highchair, sterilisers and pacifiers.

The parents who I watched while I sat on the wall at Sonny's school that morning had not done that. These were the parents of Andrea's tribe. They may not have known Andrea, but I did, and to me she was a queen of the tribe. I have a feeling I would have been in the other tribe, Elinor's tribe, had I been faced with the same choice and had I not met Sonny, Maff and Andrea. But I was most definitely not in that tribe now.

Beccy was adopted by a single woman, a Christian, who felt called to caring for the child.

## 21

## **Blow torch and matches**

While we were waiting for our tickets from Liverpool Football Club, I invited Sonny round to my house. I turned it into a birthday celebration after I received this text from Andrea:

*It's been a weird day. I always feel so overly emotional on Sonny's bday, like I don't know what to do with myself and my feelings. Every year! I don't like it. It'll pass and tomorrow I shall be normal again. So strange how we associate dates with feelings and emotions. Love to you xx*

The plan was to spend some time with Sonny while the adults had some food and drink, which, translated into Somerset, meant getting trashed.

On the back of the Thompson van is an official looking sign that says: ZOMBIE OUTBREAK RESPONSE VEHICLE. The two girls tumbled out of the vehicle, leaving Sonny in the gloom. Talulah had won an art competition and a scholarship for her new school. Delilah had grown. They brought a friend with them who skipped off after a football he saw in the hedge.

I was always torn around the Thompson family, because they were all good company, but I felt sensitive about neglecting Sonny, who at that moment was strapped into the vehicle facing the windscreen while his sisters chattered to me.

I called, 'Hi Sonny, hi Maff,' into the van. Andrea jumped out of the driving seat holding the black shoulder bag with batteries, tubes and wires, opened the back doors and activated the lift. Maff was untethering Sonny, talking quietly to him.

'All right?' he murmured. 'Let's get you over here young man.' He dipped his head to kiss him, while Andrea held the controller on the coiled wire and extended the ramp out of the back of the van. Sonny was lowered to the ground. I touched the soft hand on the arm of his chair.

'Radiator Peach,' I said. 'Good to see you.'

I have a large fire dish in my garden and I suggested Sonny and I light it 'together'. I was using 'together' in Andrea's sense, meaning just involve Sonny at any level possible. Or involve him using the sense that she found most reliable, beating sight, hearing and touch: psychic. I shooed everyone into the house to be alone with Sonny.

'You start with paper,' I said, picking up an old *Guardian*, 'and you roll it up like this,' I made it into a tube. 'You don't scrunch it, it needs to be denser than that, and you can't just chuck on an old paper without rolling the pages, as that would be too dense and the oxygen couldn't get in. A fire needs help to breathe. Like you,' I smiled. 'Then for maximum effect, we tie the tube into a knot like a doughnut.'

I then picked out some dead leaves and grasses from the basket and laid them over the paper, explaining what I was doing as I went. On top of them I placed kindling in a little tipi and on that a couple of dry split ash logs.

'That should do it,' I said, reaching for the blow torch and matches. I chose the torch for dramatic effect. And I thought holding his hand down on the match box while I struck it could go wrong, particularly with that cylinder of oxygen right behind him.

I lit it right in front of his eyes. The yellow flame made a satisfying roar as it turned blue. Andrea appeared in the doorway, possibly to check I wasn't going to send her son up in flames, but also to see this moment for Sonny, when he had some genuine interaction with a person who wasn't family, or a carer being paid to give him attention. I then got the flames licking at the paper and kindling, and soon the fire was making a promising noise.

'That sound means it's alight,' I said. 'A silent fire is a dying fire.' A crack and some sparks flew off a bit of pine. Sonny made either no reaction, or a reaction so subtle I couldn't perceive it, but I was busy not setting his feet, which were quite close to the flames, on fire.

As I rolled him back a couple of inches I said 'Never trust a man who uses firelighters. These yours?' I held up the matches and pretended to put them in his top pocket, which he didn't have. I smiled at him. I was trying to dignify him, respect him, treat him like any other young man.

'I'll remember that,' he didn't say. But I said it in my head for him.

Maff approached us across the lawn with a drink.

'How are you, Sonny? Suction? Cold? Too hot?'

'I want to get him close enough so he feels the warmth on his face,' I said.

'Okay,' said Maff, clicking off the brake and pulling him back another foot. 'I think we should be fine about here.'

I had laid on some gin, which everyone but Maff – who clutched a single can of beer all night – started drinking. The girls found some water pistols and ran round firing them at us.

'Cold?' said Maff to Sonny again. 'Suction? Want to look at the garden? Turn this way? Suction.' He stripped the packaging off a fresh straw and flicked on the pump.

We pulled up garden chairs to sit with Sonny around the fire – a truly Somerset arrangement – and then started talking some quality drunken nonsense, respecting another fine Somerset tradition.

'Let me tell you,' I said to Sonny, 'having two pairs of spectacles is like having two women.'

'Did you just say that, Guy?' Andrea said.

'Yes. Listen. I'm imparting wisdom to Sonny. If you have two or even three pairs, when you lose one, you just go and look for the second pair. You don't look hard for the original pair, right? Same with women, young man,' I said.

'Do not listen to him on that subject,' Andrea said.

A chill came in the air, so the girls went inside to watch TV leaving the young lad with us, and we wrapped our jackets tighter and moved a little closer to the bright, silent empire of burning logs on their bed of glowing ash. The little boy said to me 'Don't you know smoking is bad for you?'

I said 'No, I'd never heard that.'

He said 'I think you're drinking too much. I'm going inside.'

I watched the nipper run indoors.

Andrea draped Sonny in a leopard print stole. Sonny was so cool. He let us do anything. He never criticised or judged me badly. He was what I called fine company.

The flames were entrancing. I had used dead box plants for kindling and the remains of them crackled and burned fast and brightly. I could see the warmth on Sonny's red cheeks. He was definitely looking at this.

'Is he too close to the fire dish?' Maff said.

'Let him feel the warmth,' I said. 'Though we don't want to melt his chair, that's true.'

Our talk turned to the festival, the Glastonbury Festival, which all local people called Pilton. That was how we could tell if people were from around there. I told a story of accidentally dropping two tabs of acid, and it was soon topped by more stories of accidental and deliberate acts of excess. Sonny quietly listened in. The things that boy must have heard, because adults spoke of subjects in front of him which they would never with a different boy who had just turned sixteen. It wasn't because I thought he was dumb. It was because I thought he possessed a kind of ageless wisdom. And his judgement was always so kind and patient, however idiotic we were. Where to get the best coke, how many pills to drop and at what interval – the man was an expert, but a silent and very discreet one.

'The sunset,' Andrea said. 'Come on, Sonny,' she got up to turn him to face where the orange disc was dropping between a neighbour's barn and a tree.

I was quite drunk. 'Look at the sunset – dramatic and bright,' I said. 'Isn't that a thing to see?' I squeezed his knuckle-less hand.

'Isn't that magical?' Andrea said.

We both turned to Sonny as we cooed over the view. I wasn't entirely sure if Sonny was really looking at the tree, which now seemed burnished with fire. When I glanced at him I was worried he was looking at the grass, or my neighbour's wall.

An hour later we were still sitting staring at the embers, still feeling the heat.

'Look at Sonny,' I said. 'I wonder what he's thinking.'

Andrea laughed and said, 'sometimes I don't think there's anything going on in that head of his.' But she said it in such a way that the state of empty-headedness seemed ideal, a state of grace.

But it was a pretty big statement for her to make. I put it down to the booze and smoke and an attempt at light-hearted banter, but she nudged the doubts which were stirring in my mind. I remembered the ease with which we steered Sonny away from the match with Brentford, and his absence of apparent joy at the prospect of seeing Manchester United.

For a devoted sixteen-year-old Liverpool supporter there was nothing more exciting than seeing a Liverpool versus Man U game. But I hadn't picked up any signals that Sonny was even aware we were talking about it.

I felt in my pocket for my notebook to jot these thoughts down and realised I had left it somewhere in the house, I couldn't remember where. In the early days it was always open on my knee. I guess it was a sign I had stopped expecting breakthrough events, that I had nothing more to note down about Sonny because he had nothing more to give me. The initial determination on all sides (especially mine) to push Sonny to perform a miracle had slackened, even petered out.

I turned my attention to my campaign to convince Maff that I was a genuine Liverpool Football supporter and not making the claim to ingratiate myself.

'You're not from Liverpool, how come you're such a devoted supporter?' I asked him.

'I grew up in that golden period for the club in the 80s. When we were European champions with Kenny Dalglish, and Graeme Souness.'

I smiled carefully, aware of my precarious record.

'But the player who really affected me was John Barnes,' Maff added.

I could nod with full confidence at this reference because John Barnes was a player famous not just for his football skills, but his handsome looks and his unusual, for the time, brown skin. He was basically the first truly brilliant and famous black British footballer of the modern era.

'I remember seeing a photo of him in a tabloid in the supermarket when I was shopping with my mum,' Maff said. 'I didn't get on so well with my dad and I suppose I was looking for a father figure – somehow John Barnes filled that gap. I became obsessed by him. I had posters, and football cards of him at home. He was a kind of god.'

'I used to have to watch Liverpool games as a kid,' Andrea said. 'On Saturdays we always went round to my cousin's house who supported Liverpool, so I ended up sitting there watching it.'

As the fire diminished, we drew closer to watch the embers glow. Maff checked his watch. Sonny had to get home, and the van had to be loaded. In the gathering darkness they pushed him across the dewy grass. I waved as Sonny ascended on the tail lift of the van, and seeing their tail-lights disappear up the lane, returned to the fire dish to contemplate his future.

## 22

## **Bliss amongst the crowd**

I learnt something important when Pilton, the festival, came around. My home is in the small village adjacent to the small city that sprang up as a result of the revels. Living so close to the festival site, I sensed the excitement on the roads and the adrenalin in the air in the days that preceded its start, when 300,000 ravers pitched up on the other side of a metal fence at the bottom of my garden for four days of musical and pharmaceutical excess.

It was obviously exactly the kind of event which Maff and Andrea adored: their generosity of spirit was perfect to spread the love and bliss amongst the crowd. They were both from Somerset. Its people knew how to party. At a professional level. Have you ever seen Berliners party? Well, give them a couple of shots, a pinger or two, and run 1000 volts through the lot of them and you have something of the energy of the Somerset festival tribe in full cry.

But Pilton was not Sonny territory. The first breathtaking view of the multicoloured city of tents, stages and crowds glimpsed between trees from a steep uneven track would totally rock Sonny, but not in the right way. At the bottom of the lane, in the middle of the festival site, the ground of the valley floor was flatter but strewn with obstacles like flag poles, litter bins, guy ropes, and sleeping punters. Dust would interfere with Sonny's air intake and, if rain fell, the chair would get mired in the famous glutinous mud. Punters staggered and lurched around, blind to what was in front of them.

There was also an absence of power sockets and very little chance of getting Sonny out of the festival in an emergency; like, for instance, if we had departed Frome in such a rush of excitement and discovered in the middle of a seething mass of people that we had left both spare batteries for his ventilator back at home. If that happened, Sonny could die. That was not a risk worth taking.

So it was agreed he couldn't go. I didn't think he minded that much. Why would Sonny enjoy Pilton? His taste was for sitting down and talking with friends – two activities impossible at the festival because the music was too loud to converse over and there were 300,000 people and fifty-seven seats, although he did bring his own.

I never thought Sonny was that into music, though Andrea insisted he was. With characteristic modesty, Maff quietly played a sweet guitar, and Andrea sang with the voice of an angel who had been smoking American Spirit roll-ups for half of eternity, but Sonny still looked uninterested.

'He loves his music,' Andrea shouted at me as she turned up the volume on some 90s banger called 'Where Love Lives' which she had danced to in her twenties. 'Don't you Sonny?'

So when the festival came round, Andrea rang me and said 'Come and see me and Sonny on Wednesday, Maff will be over on the site. He's going alone.' She sounded a little deflated, despite not making a big deal out of it.

I drove over, leaving behind me the crawling traffic, the eerie glow of a floodlit night sky and the growing perturbation of the Glastonbury Festival.

As Andrea answered the door she said in a sing song voice, 'Oh my god I am so disappointed.'

With a click I unscrewed the top of a bottle of wine, filled two glasses and wedged in beside Sonny.

This is how I assessed the situation: Sonny, listening to all the conversations between Maff and Andrea, knew exactly why Maff wasn't there and Andrea was. He didn't look guilty, but he seemed grateful. His mum had stayed to look after him.

'You're taking it pretty well,' I said to Andrea.

'It's what it is and I cannot change anything, so I am accepting it,' she smiled, then wailed 'Waaah!'

I topped up her glass and mine.

'Look at these,' she scrolled her photos. Sonny was in the school café by the door as a couple of students walked past in the foreground. 'He's meeting and greeting,' Andrea said. I nodded. 'He gets the washing up to do,' she said. And I nodded at that too out of sheer love for her and Sonny. Quite how Sonny could tackle a pile of dirty crockery and cutlery was not explained, but nor in that moment did it need to be. I was leaning into it. That's what we all did when Andrea was around. 'Work experience,' Andrea added.

There was a sound that some of my friends made, I think they were all female, when looking at kittens in a basket or cute babies in basinets. It went 'Awwwww.' It was not a phoneme which I myself could ever enunciate. I don't know why. It was just too soppy for a real man like me.

But inside my head, and maybe my heart, when Andrea talked about Sonny doing work experience, and I thought about Sonny going out into the harsh world, I heard a long soft Awwwww. Andrea said, 'Let's have more wine.'

Not far away, over the hill, one of the biggest and most beguiling parties on earth was warming up its engines. All Andrea's friends were on site, and all of them I knew for certain would have loved to see Andrea dancing and laughing among them. But the three of us made a fine evening of it in Frome. We found a thread of conversation and teased it out between us, pulling it from the ball of thought and experience, and plaiting it with memories and stories.

Always an expert in the now (as she would have said), Andrea created and warmed the bubble that the three of us found ourselves inside. She kept up lively talk, deftly keeping Sonny in the chat, like casually knocking a tennis ball against a wall so it dropped back to us. He was totally reliable; it was we who occasionally had to run off and get a stray ball. You couldn't get it past Sonny.

At one point she said, 'Did you hear that Mr T? Guy actually believes in gravity! Have you ever heard such a silly thing? He doesn't even believe in magic, or parallel universes! I'm surprised he can cross the road.'

The thought of the party over the hill receded. The festival stopped being a place we weren't at, and the lounge of the house in Frome became the only place to be that night. Andrea and Sonny had transformed FOMO – Fear Of Missing Out – into FOBI - Fun Of Being In.

That night Sonny was incontrovertibly present, even alert, as we talked and drank way past his bedtime. Anxiety evaporated, we relaxed, feeling strong, stable and secure. And Sonny had occasioned it simply by being present and listening to us. Can you hear someone listening? That night I most definitely could. Understanding Sonny was a kind of magic. Andrea taught me that. And although I drew the line at tree faeries and crystals, I believed in that magic.

In a gap in the conversation, I think after Andrea said, 'You know we're all from another planet, don't you?' I heard/felt/

sensed Sonny fill the silence with unvoiced thoughts: 'Thank you,' he said. 'Mum. Thank you for not leaving me. Thank you for not deserting me, tonight, or ever. And thank you, Guy, for keeping us company and making it fun.'

I was definitely in the right place that night. I learnt life was on the side of the festival wall you found yourself. FOBI. The fun of being in. I learnt about that from Sonny and Andrea.

## 23

### Stuttering and failing

A week after the festival, I arrived at the house to see Sonny in his usual spot in his throne outside his bedroom. Fox went barmy with me at the door, barking and jumping up on my white trousers.

'How shot is your memory, Fox?' I said as I brushed her aside. 'It's me, we've only met fifty times.'

I went straight to Sonny. I sat down and touched his arm, as soft as a broad bean pod.

'Have you told him the news?' I asked Andrea who was round the corner in the kitchen.

'No, we thought we'd leave it to you.'

I got out my phone and opened an email.

'Dear Guy,' I said, 'Thank you for contacting Liverpool Football Club. Please accept our sincere apologies for any confusion caused. We have arranged tickets for Sonny to come to the Wolves game on *10/09/22* (this may be subject to change). We will arrange three tickets that will be charged at a concession rate, we will be in contact the week of the game to arrange this. If I can be of any further assistance, Guy, then please get back in touch. Thank you for your continued support. Kind regards, Daniel. Ticketing Services. Liverpool Football Club.'

'That's ten weeks away,' said Andrea. 'We're going to Liverpool!'

I had thought that Andrea might not want to come, but after a glance at Maff I knew she was on the trip.

From the way the subject was avoided I sensed that progress on the Eye-Gaze had been slow and difficult for Sonny.

I said, 'Is he able to tell his friends at school on the Eye-Gaze that he's going to Anfield?' I asked.

I privately thought that after years of listening to Andrea the vocabulary he needed was not available on the screen. It had icons for things like the toilet, the light, a potato chip, a dog and a baby. But the words Sonny needed to join in with Andrea were things like aura, wood nymph, leprechaun, time traveller, alien and parallel universe.

Andrea said. 'You can do that, can't you Mr T?'

But later, when I watched Sonny in front of the Eye-Gaze screen, stuttering and failing at even the most basic linguistic communication with the cursor dashing around looking terrified of something, I realised that there was no chance that Sonny could string together the words and sentences required to tell his school mates and teachers about the trip to Anfield. After months on the machine he couldn't reliably get the machine to croak out the word 'football'.

## 24

## **Random bunch of losers**

Liverpool had not had a good start to the season. After narrowly failing to win the League and two cups last season, hopes were high for the first few matches. But a sequence of losses and draws had sunk us down the table. Over the summer we had sold Sadio Mané, the Senegalese striker who we thought was merely a replaceable cog in a winning machine but who had turned out to be the power pack. Without Mané we were a random bunch of losers. We had just lost *4-1* to Napoli. And to make matters worse, Wolves had signed a devilish new striker called Diego.

I was genuinely concerned that I was finally going to get Sonny to his first game at Anfield only to see them beaten by Wolverhampton Wanderers, hardly top-drawer opposition. I already feared Sonny was harbouring doubts about my credibility, and now I worried we were heading for a big disappointment. I had been talking about this match, and the inevitable triumph it would be, for weeks, building it up and describing its details.

Sonny, Maff, Andrea and I were travelling in the bus. Carers Zoe and Nuala were going by train and meeting us at the hotel. I had four rooms booked: Sonny's, the carers', Maff and Andrea's, and mine.

Andrea texted me:

Soooo, just had a chat with the hotel about Sonny. They've allocated a connecting room with Nuala and Zoe which I think is sensible and interconnected room next to the town house (I presume is yours?), all on level 4. I've sorted out the oxygen delivery and the front desk were incredibly helpful. So nice. They've also agreed to me bringing a blender for Sonny's room.

The restaurant - bit of a different story here. The lady I spoke to wasn't so helpful. They will blend some of his food but not all of it because they use their blenders for other things. I think we will have to blend in the room which isn't a prob anyways. I think she was saying we cannot take our own food into the restaurant. We'll see about that! Sonny has what he needs to have whatever anyone else thinks. Love you. *2 more sleeps* 💤 😴 Sent from my Android.

On the Friday morning we were due to travel, I turned on the radio to discover that the Queen had died at Balmoral. I didn't feel strongly either way. My mind was on the mission. The house was chaotic. The lounge had disappeared under all the boxes and suitcases.

'The Queen's dead,' Andrea said.

'Might the match be cancelled?' asked Maff, scrolling for information. 'Out of respect or something?'

'I don't respect her that much,' Andrea said.

'We're going,' I said. 'Full speed ahead. There are fifty thousand people going to the match tomorrow, they can't possibly cancel it.'

Andrea and Maff were checking over the equipment.

'Alder Hey is the nearest intensive care,' Andrea said, conversationally, the way you might say, 'There's a Wetherspoons near the ground,' reminding me that with Sonny we were never far from catastrophe.

'Ventilator *1*, ventilator *2*,' said Andrea, flicking open cardboard boxes. 'How many suction machines do we need?'

'His spare in a box and one over there,' said Maff.

'Let's take three,' said Andrea.

'Good call,' said Maff, the supreme team player.

'Why three?' I asked.

'In case they break down,' said Maff. 'Out of all that kit, the suction machines are the things that go wrong.'

Maff was giving Sonny a quick dash of physio before running the straw into the tracheostomy. When we heard the gurgling sound Maff said, 'Ahh, there we go. Catch the phlegm.'

It was like a big cough, but of course Sonny couldn't cough so it had to be done for him.

Maff looked at me anxiously. 'The season is going so badly,' he said quietly.

'Two trachies,' Andrea called out.

'Check.'

'Full batteries for ventilator. Lasts for four hours. You have to keep an eye on it 'cos they just go.'

'So, one battery should cover the whole match,' I said.

'We'll take two full ones so if something goes wrong we're covered,' said Maff.

I suppressed an image of a crowd-crushing disaster, with Maff and me trying to protect Sonny from being trampled in its midst.

'Splints,' said Andrea.

'Check.' I counted eight large cardboard boxes and four long thin ones for the splints that reached into his lungs.

'Monkey,' said Andrea, holding up Sonny's soft toy.

'Check,' said Maff.

Fox was running around sensing the mood.

'Finn's looking after Fox,' Andrea said. 'I still haven't found the hairdryer ... just have to do without it.'

## Sonny

Sonny sat barefoot in the middle of the preparations wearing a Liverpool shirt, camo trousers and a Liverpool cap. I gave him a look which said 'See? I said I'd get you to Anfield and that is exactly what we are doing.' He started beeping.

'What's that?'

'Nothing. Water in the tube,' Andrea said, moving the breathing tube. 'We've only got one SPO2,' she said. 'Two humidifiers. Two vents. Eye-Gaze and stand.'

'Check,' said Maff.

'Let's start loading the bus.'

Maff went out, slid back the side door and opened the back doors, lowering the lift. Sonny sat in the middle of the activity. What a joy of a child, I said to myself. No moaning, no complaining, no messing around and getting in the way. Just quietly sitting still until it was time to head north.

As Maff released the brakes on Sonny's chair and guided him towards the door and the packed van, his phone pinged with a text.

He read: 'Out of respect for Her late Majesty Queen Elizabeth II all Premier League matches are being called off.' I looked up at Sonny, who was pointed with strong intention at the open door.

'Oh no,' said Maff. 'The match is off because of the Queen.'

I thought, *How the hell am I going to explain this to Sonny?* On so many occasions, Sonny had seen his siblings and others leave through that door in a state of excitement to do something from which he was excluded. Here, at last, was the day when he was going to be the one going on an outing. And yet the adults were trooping out to the van to retrieve all the boxes and cases they had just loaded.

I sat down beside Sonny. I stared at him and put my hand over his.

'I'm afraid there's been a fuck up,' I explained, 'and we can't go to watch the lads play today.'

I thought I saw alarm on his little face.

'I know I know I know,' I said.

'Get me a drink,' said Andrea with her head in the fridge.

'This is the best argument for Britain becoming a republic I have ever seen,' Maff said.

We got the kit in from the van and I tried to explain to Sonny about the monarchy, and how when the head of it died football matches couldn't be played. My view is that he listened to me and thought *Do you really think I'm going to fall for that? An old lady at the end of her life dies, and we can't watch footy? That is such a pathetic lame excuse. Why not just tell me straight you don't want to go to the match, you've changed your mind, or you don't want to be seen with me in public. Just say it, Guy.*

## 25

## It's strange

It is not my habit to put words into people's mouths. I have not speculated about Maff or Andrea's thoughts. I am not a mind reader. But I couldn't stop doing it with Sonny. Every time I was in his presence my brain filled with what sounded like him talking. It was as though he had a voice, which I could hear. You think that sounds bonkers, wait for what came next.

When people asked how I communicated with Sonny I said, 'I really don't know. It's strange. Unaccountable. Maybe I am making it all up, but it seems like it's coming from him,' shrugged, smiled and shook my head.

Then I came upon *The Telepathy Tapes*. This was a podcast made in America by a woman called Ky Dickens which advanced the proposition that non-verbal autistic people could communicate telepathically. At the beginning of each episode she said:

*For decades, a very specific group of people have been claiming telepathy is happening. Nobody has believed them. Nobody has listened to them. But on this podcast, we do.*

## It's strange

She had been reaching *100,000* downloads for a couple of years when the show went viral and got *15* million downloads. That was a sign to me that something was going on.

But before I sat down with *The Telepathy Tapes*, I watched a documentary called *Tell Them You Love Me*.

## 26

## **Tell Them You Love Me**

This full-length documentary was about a young American who was non-verbal and had cerebral palsy. I watched it on my laptop beside my open Sonny notebook.

The disabled man was called Derrick. He could walk, but he didn't have good control of his arms and hands. My initial assessment, ten minutes into the film, was that on the disability spectrum he wasn't far from Sonny. His mum, a likeable woman called Daisy, had to feed him, and he used a nappy at thirty years of age. He grunted and moaned, and communication looked murky. I noticed Daisy occasionally singing, even though Derrick didn't seem to comprehend it. It was like an additional loving effort she was prepared to make to get through to her son. Familiar territory for me.

Derrick's older brother, John, also seemed protective and loving. 'What is going on in your head, Derrick? To me that was the great mystery,' he said to camera.

I shifted in my seat. This was the first time I had ever seen anything close to the household in Frome.

John had attended a lecture by the Director of Philosophy of Disability Studies at Rutgers University, where he was a postgraduate. The professor was a woman called Anna Stubblefield. She was a well turned out academic with short hair and no-nonsense eyes, exuding rational calm. Anna's mum, who we briefly saw, wore a t-shirt that said LABELS ARE FOR JARS NOT PEOPLE.

'It's not the impairment, it's the environment that creates impairments,' Anna said to the camera. She advanced the theory that spoken language was not the marker of intelligence, and her work had focused on helping non-verbal patients communicate with the aid of a special keyboard which was called a Neo.

The viewer was then swept to Australia and introduced to a woman in her thirties with dystonia and autism, quite unable to control her movements or talk, whose arm was supported by a carer to help her type on a Neo. Having never uttered a word in her life, it turned out this woman could spell. She typed the sentence: thank you for giving me a voice. As I began to type my mind woke up.

Anna was an advocate of this technique, which they called facilitated communication, and lectured that it was capable of unlocking the sealed box in which many non-verbal patients dwelled.

John introduced Anna to his brother, Derrick, saying that he wondered if he could be helped.

Anna put Derrick in front of some cards with images on them, like a cat and a fork, asked him point to one, and watched Derrick fail to do so. Anna said, 'You can see how hard he works to try to have the least bit of control over his arm.'

I immediately thought about Sonny's Eye-Gaze sessions, and how difficult it had been for Sonny to control his eye movements and the cursor.

But then she said, 'I started with an initial bit of support on his elbow and then he could select which picture he wanted.' And sure enough, when Anna said dog, Derrick, with his elbow supported by Anna, pointed at the dog.

Derrick graduated to picking out letters on the Neo. It turned out Derrick could also spell. A distant alarm that rang far away in the back of my head was soon drowned out by the thudding hooves of the cavalry coming over the horizon. Derrick, though mobile, had a lot in common with Sonny. His impenetrable expressions and his wandering eyes for a start.

Anna and Derrick worked together on the Neo, refining Derrick's typing skills. 'I was keeping his fingers folded down so his index finger was isolated. I asked him to point to letters. And it was like the porch lights went on.'

By the end of the year, Derrick was writing sentences and having conversations. For instance, he once said, or wrote, to Anna, 'Nobody told me you were running late so I was not sure you were coming.' Which is an astonishingly sophisticated remark from someone who, a few months earlier, only produced grunts and moans. His brother said, 'It somewhat confirmed what I already knew.'

If Derrick could *spell* (and understand tenses), there was a real chance, I now believed, that we might get some communication with Sonny. Anna and Derrick proved that what Andrea (and I) was thinking was not outlandish. She confirmed my belief in Andrea's world, and in Sonny's abilities.

A few months later, Derrick was enrolled on a course at Rutgers University studying African American literature. Anna sat beside him, providing 'communication support', and soon Derrick was asking questions in class and turning in essays. According to Anna, Derrick was 'a really intellectual guy.' Derrick graduated onto the speaking circuit and started giving lectures.

I was fascinated by Derrick's transformation and obviously wondered whether something similar could be done for Sonny. I didn't think Sonny was ever going to knock out *1000* words on James Baldwin, which for Derrick was a doddle, but this made me think that Sonny could at least say *Hello* and *I love you, Mum.*

But there was a shot in the movie, of Derrick's hand being supported as he typed, which reminded me of the day Zoe and I had played with the remote-controlled car with Sonny. Zoe and I had lifted Sonny's hand onto the remote to make the car shoot across the floor. But I remembered that, although it looked like Sonny was touching the controls, it was actually Zoe and I doing it. We had just pretended it was Sonny.

Back in the film, the story took an unpredicted turn: Anna fell in love with Derrick, and Derrick typed *I love you too* back to her.

'He asked me to kiss him,' Anna said into the camera, without a trace of anxiety, which was surely the emotion uppermost in the minds of everyone watching. I felt distinctly queasy as she described in excruciating detail how she had sex with Derrick, who of course still had great difficulty with movement and was unable to talk.

If that wasn't enough, a second development leapt from the screen: Derrick's mum and brother, who I had grown to like and respect, thinking how similar they were to Andrea and Maff, admitted that they couldn't make the Neo work.

They were unable to talk to Derrick on the typing machine.

'Two words would come out of it, but it didn't make any sense,' admitted John.

Radiator peach.

The more Derrick talked while Anna 'supported' – yes, I now have to use quotation marks – his hand to find the letters, the more extraordinary were the things that emerged. He announced that he no longer liked Daisy's home cooking or the gospel music he had listened to all his life, but was a vegetarian with a penchant for Mozart. He even preferred wine over beer.

Plus, he announced via the keyboard that he wanted to leave home and move into supervised housing.

This was all explained over a shot of Derrick's black hand being held at the wrist by a white woman's hand while he touched the letters. My eyes were closely examining the grip of the woman's fingers.

Anna also had announcements: she wanted to leave her husband and marry Derrick. This came out when she had told a stunned Daisy and John that she had already had sex with Derrick.

This admission was too much for everyone. John and Daisy informed the university, and the Dean suspended Anna and called in the Police, who charged the professor with sexual offences.

When the court case came round, an expert witness explained that throughout the whole period of Derrick's transformation it had been Anna, not Derrick, using the keyboard.

'It was bogus,' said John, who was clearly and rightfully angry.

The expert witness had designed an ingenious test in which he showed a different image to the patient and the supporting carer but made them think it was the same picture. In every example, the patient typed what the 'facilitator' saw, rather than the patient. It was absolutely certain that the patient was being influenced by the person holding their hand. Influence was the word they used. To me, it looked like the patient was being controlled by the carer.

After independent tests, the court was informed that Derrick was not able to communicate with any devices of any kind.

Anna Stubblefield was sentenced to 6-12 months. Derrick's life as an independent, Burgundy-drinking classical music devotee was scrapped, and he went back to his old ways.

A friend of Anna Stubblefield said towards the end of the film, 'Anna was having conversations with herself and I don't know where you would go with that.'

I paused the film, leant back in my chair, let out the lungful of air which had apparently got trapped there, and reflected on my own interactions with Sonny.

In Derrick's case, his entire identity had been a comprehensive act of projection by Anna, who had got everybody to go along with it. What were her motives? The distasteful romantic and sexual elements turned her into a nasty predator. It was crazy that nobody had stopped her sooner. I suspect everybody around her had cut her a lot of slack because she was a renowned, and white, academic, and Derrick, Daisy and John were black and not rich.

The snow globe I stood in beside Sonny – that insulated, magical world – had been given a good shake by *Tell Them You Love Me*. My doubts about his lack of cognitive ability frightened me. I felt like my heart had gone into reverse and was pumping blood the wrong way round my body.

Had I vastly overestimated what was going on inside Sonny? Had I been looking into his face and making it all up?

Sonny had been unable to pass on my message to Maff about going to the football match. I hadn't mentioned that to you, patient reader. Why?

Why had I been so confident that the cumulative effect of his eyebrows wiggling, eyes rolling and skin blushing were meaningful?

After seeing Derrick and Anna's sorry story, I feared I was lying to myself. And by extension, to you, my tolerant reader. I knew my motives were pure – unlike Anna's, whose motives remain a sordid and twisted mystery – but I had not yet disentangled them. During the weeks away from the Thompson family, I started doing that.

From my first meeting with Sonny, I had felt deficient; not seeing what the others around Sonny seemed to be noticing. When they said what his favourite colour was, or that he liked to listen to the Libertines or that he was saying Yes or No, I thought the fault lay in me that I couldn't read him.

The documentary was not just bad news, but it was *like* bad news too, in that it had a habit of disappearing from my mind from time to time, only to return with a sharper intensity when I suddenly remembered what had happened. I would wake in the morning, or be taking a walk up the Tor and counting my blessings, before it all came back to me that I had this horrible new reality in my life: of Sonny not being Sonny.

I had been knocking at the Sonny door, telling you, kind and patient reader, to stand beside me and wait for it to be opened so we could all be there when Sonny appeared. But now I had turned the handle and was about to push open the door I feared there wasn't even a house behind it.

Two films played in my mind: *Tell Them You Love Me*, and *Guy's Encounters With Sonny*, which featured me picking through the past to see if I had fallen for the Stubblefield delusion (without the sex offences).

A scene from my personal doc was when I broke the news of the Queen's death and the cancellation of the football match. Had I really noticed 'alarm' cross Sonny's face, as I had written in my notebook? How did, how could, Sonny show alarm? He moved his eyebrows. He looked to the side, and I got the impression of anxiety. But how? Moving his eyebrows and his eyes like that was also the expression for happiness, for the simple reason that that was all he could move. When I wrote alarm I was, like the Facilitated Communicators in the other movie, influencing, leading Sonny. An echoey judicial voice sounded in my head: I put it to you, Guy Kennaway, that you were not reading Sonny's face, that you were making up his emotions to suit your manipulative and dishonest narrative.

I remembered nodding and smiling when Andrea told me that Sonny was doing work experience at his school. He was 'meeting and greeting' in the café. She showed me a photograph of him at the entrance.

He wasn't meeting and greeting. The people around him were, and we wanted him to meet and greet. Of course we did. But the truth is he was sitting motionless and expressionless in his chair as the world went on around him.

It hadn't even been hidden from me. The very first time I met Sonny I noticed Andrea and Zoe had trouble distinguishing a yes from a no. It was about whether he wanted a suction. I wrote about it and even made a joke about it. But twenty minutes after meeting them, I was already being swept through the doors and down the aisle into the church of Sonny.

I had bottled up my doubts, jammed in the cork, and pretended I spoke Sonny. Fake it to make it, is the phrase used for this flawed process. Well, it's either flawed or complete nonsense. Using it, I convinced myself Sonny was communicating with me. But the words I was ascribing to him were all from my own imagination. I made him say what I would have said in his place (not that I actually knew what that was). And, more importantly, the words I wanted him to say.

Radiator Peach was one of Sonny's first utterances, and a good case in point. The phrase was both bleak and promising. It could be read as evocative and playful, or as meaningless. The two words stood exactly atop the enigma of Sonny Thompson.

Radiator Peach. A full and complex phrase, or devoid of meaning?

The new reality, that I worried Sonny was empty, felt like a monumental betrayal of Andrea and Maff, who had led me into this extraordinary world where their child was a fully sentient person, who only those blessed with some indefinable power could understand. That was how it felt. But that whole world was under threat, and it meant I didn't only see Sonny differently, but had to revise my opinion of Andrea, Maff, all of them.

So I sat at home, avoiding the house in Frome, and wondering what I was going to do generally with them, and particularly with this book.

Many times people had said to me, when I told them about Sonny, 'Isn't it a bit sad to keep him alive if he has no quality of life? Isn't it a waste of valuable NHS resources which could be used for curable children? And how must it be for him, unable to move or talk, spending all day in a nappy being fed through a tube?' I had always countered indignantly that Sonny was a beautiful and playful human being, with a shining soul and a full, if wonky, consciousness.

But what if I had made all that up? What if they were, at least to some degree, right?

## 27

### The Telepathy Tapes

While I was avoiding the house in Frome, I took the opportunity to do more research. It was then that I listened to *The Telepathy Tapes*. The snow globe that had been tipped upside down by the documentary was picked up and given another vigorous shake.

This American podcast advanced the proposition that all non-speaking autistic people were telepathic. They could communicate with verbal people without language, and talk to other autistic people over huge distances and spend time with each other at a place they called The Hill, which existed in a different dimension.

The presenter, Ky Dickens, a determined woman from the mid-West who did not have autistic children of her own, flew around America to meet autistic kids who claimed to have the power to read minds. A girl called Mia was blindfolded while her mum was shown words and numbers on cards. The cards were put away, the blindfold removed, and Mia then correctly identified all the numbers and images.

But to make herself understood, Mia, like most of the other autistic people in *The Telepathy Tapes*, was using some kind of facilitated communication, like Derrick and the professor. It was explained in a new way to me. Whereas Anna had claimed she had no input, and the words were all Derrick's, Ky Dickinson used the metaphor of a cello and a bow. Both were doing something; the facilitator and the non-verbal person. But the words were the true thoughts of the autistic. She said it was like the hands on the shoulder of a child learning to ride a bicycle. After a bit, they were not holding the child up but just giving them confidence to ride on two wheels themselves.

There were enough extraordinary examples of these children and young adults communicating with family members and carers to attract 15 million downloads. And I didn't believe all those listeners were scoffing.

I thought hard about whether Sonny was reading my mind and, in turn, putting thoughts into it. What if he was reading my mind? The poor lad. That was something else he would be unlikely to recover from.

I listened to the full eight hours of *The Telepathy Tapes* podcast, and by the end was convinced that some non-verbal autistic children were capable of communication that could not be explained by any science I knew about.

This may have been the reason I kept writing down Sonny's thoughts. I was hearing them.

Everything was all right. Sonny was alive and well in there, chatting to us all. With a vibrant social life on the Hill.

I started looking around the internet for what people made of *The Telepathy Tapes,* and it didn't take long to find an article that, while not pouring a bucket of cold water over it, blasted it with an icy spray of scepticism. And, no sooner had I read that, I came across another person who swore her child was telepathic.

There was no end to research about what non-verbal people were capable or not capable of. Everybody had a story, and a theory. As soon as the snow settled in my glass dome, I would be given another shake. I existed in a blizzard of claim, counterclaim, refutation and reassertion criss-crossing around me.

The only thing that was clear was that all these theories were born from the love and care and maybe desperation of parents and friends who wanted to make some sense which they could live with. Otherwise, it was too terrifying loving a child like Sonny.

## 28

## **Lifting the bread**

I did finally drag myself round to the house in Frome where Maff and Andrea welcomed me with their customary warmth. I felt like somebody considering betrayal.

The two of them busied themselves around the house. Andrea was soon saying, 'Okay darling, so you pick them up and drop them at Julie's and I'll pick them and Ben up from her and bring them back and give them tea here ...'

I sat on the wide leather arm of the family sofa beside Sonny, and looked into his face. He was on the Eye-Gaze. Was it a hopeless enterprise or a lifeline?

I had wondered if the lack of progress would have consigned the screen to its black travel case, but lack of progress with Sonny meant more belief was needed. And who knew, maybe he was making progress, even if it was too small to notice. Maybe all he needed was more time and the right facilitator.

He lolled back in his throne, staring at a point a metre in front of him while I searched his impenetrable face and distant eyes for meaning. Deep into that lovely, moon-like face, I looked for a message. But none came. None that I could discern.

I sighed, stood up and went to get a mug of tea.

His deep-sea gaze must have passed over the screen as I left because the croaking computer-generated voice said, '*13:32.*'

'He likes to tell the time,' Maff said.

Then the voice said, 'clock alarm, light, fan, selfie.'

The machine sounded like Stephen Hawking.

'*13:54,*' it said. Then, '*13:55.*'

I felt sad, and said, 'He likes things that are not emotional. He must be watching the number change,' because I couldn't say what was on my mind. It felt too cruel to pour cold water over the whole Sonny-can-talk-if-you-know-how-to-listen thing. Cruel to Andrea, to Maff, to the girls and the carers. And it was cruel to Sonny if I was wrong and he was listening. And of course I could be wrong, though how, it was getting harder for me to see.

'I think he just likes to tell the time,' Andrea said.

Unlike Anna Stubblefield, who interfered with what Derrick produced, Andrea just made sense of Sonny's strange utterances.

I nodded. One thing was for certain, and you couldn't say it about Derrick, who was always ducking and weaving and moaning and groaning, Sonny didn't seem restless or frustrated.

Maff said, 'What time is it, Sonny?'

Sonny didn't answer.

We all laughed. I'm not certain why we laughed. It definitely was funny. I guess we had all brushed up against the dark frightening truth.

I asked how things were going. Andrea said that with Sonny turning sixteen the transition from child to adult services in the Council Care Service would begin.

'Is that a good thing?' I asked.

'There's more money in child services, but it will be great not being monitored and overlooked all the time. They leave you alone. We won't constantly have meetings with dietitians, or the whole professional team: respiratory, cardiac, orthopaedics, CGT, CHCT, SALT, neurology, physios, OT, clinical genetics ...'

'I'm going to need my notebook,' I said.

'Yes,' she said, 'there are a lot of them.'

'Are they still objecting to you feeding Sonny the same food as you all eat?'

'They want him on the formula,' Andrea said, 'which makes him vomit.'

After the whirring sound of the blender, Andrea brought through dinner. We ate grilled sardines, home-made quiche and basmati rice, with Sonny's portion blended and sucked up into the syringe with a pull of the plunger.

'You know I said we were doing more tests on Sonny, genetic tests?' Andrea said, as Maff pushed the food down the tube into Sonny's tummy. 'Well, we got the results.'

'Like a diagnosis?' I said.

'The doctor actually said to us, "Am I supposed to find another diagnosis?" We said what do you mean? He said, "according to Sonny's notes, he was diagnosed in *2012* with Spinal Muscular Atrophy".'

I tried to process this astonishing bit of intelligence.

'But you never told me that,' I said.

'We didn't know,' Andrea said.

'But didn't the doctor say he told you in *2012*?'

Maff said, 'I looked back through the paperwork and couldn't find any mention of it.'

That seemed to be beyond credibility, and there was something in his manner which made me wonder if there was something he wasn't telling me, or for that matter, Andrea. Like he had shielded us for our protection, and Sonny's protection. Surely the diagnosis would have come up in one of the many meetings they attended with health professionals? But they both denied knowing about it. They had either forgotten it or had never taken it on board to start with, or it revealed a shocking shortcoming in the NHS. I favoured the second theory. I always thought that Andrea considered a diagnosis a box which she wouldn't be able to magic Sonny out of.

'There are four types of SMA,' Maff explained. 'One – from birth. Two – from *12* months. Three – from *18* months. And four – older children. I have been reading about the symptoms since hearing this and I think it's what Sonny has.'

'So, the doctor said he had told you, but neither of you remembered?'

'It was not on any paperwork,' Maff repeated.

'I think it was missed,' said Andrea. 'Fell through a crack in the NHS.'

'Does this change things?' I asked.

'Extensive studies and pharmaceutical trials have made really good progress with it, if treated early enough,' Maff said.

There was a pause.

'One lad had a million-pound injection on the NHS,' Maff added.

'I don't know where the information went,' Andrea said. 'I don't know if he's missed the boat.'

She got up and gave him some physio and suction until he gurgled.

'There you go,' she said.

Back at home, I got on the NHS website to research Spinal Muscular Atrophy. It was as Maff had described, but he had either failed to mention or not known that it was not connected to mental development. It accounted for the floppy body and inability to breathe but not the difficulties with communication. It clearly said that a reduced life expectancy came with the SMA package.

## 29

## Ticketing services

An email from Liverpool Football Club Ticketing services arrived.

*28 Feb 2023*

*Hi Guy,*

*Thanks for taking my call.*

*I have now booked you in for the Manchester United fixture on 4th March as discussed.*

*I will be in contact with you in due course.*

*Kind regards.*

*Shelley D.*

Manchester United. That was a break. Just when I most needed it. Thank god for the monarchy. United at Anfield. It was the big one. One of the most celebrated fixtures in world football. Maff would be so excited. I certainly was.

I called Andrea.

'I've got some good news,' I said. 'We've got Man U.'

'Have you?' she said in a hollow voice.

'What's wrong, Andrea?' I asked.

'We've had a bad week. Sonny's been ill. His breathing. He has been very full, his lungs. We nearly took him to intensive care but I didn't want to make the wrong call because they might not let him out. In the end we saw it through ourselves with antibiotics, but we are both exhausted and Maff has had to take the week off, so we are short of money as he doesn't get paid. I'm sorry not to be positive. We are at the end of our tethers; we just need to rest.'

I heard in her voice the seconds, minutes, hours, days, weeks, months and years of looking after Sonny pressing on her soul. The relentless emotional and physical demands of having him in her care weighed down on her, flattening her voice to a monotone, squeezing out the joy, and the fight.

'What about this match?' she asked.

'It's in March, so we've got a bit of time, let's hope Sonny's stronger by then.'

I went over to see her the next day. Maff was at work. Andrea had lost a lot of weight and looked drained. Her bonny cheeks were sunken and the sparkling eyes were dull.

'He's been having quite a bit of physio,' she said as we walked through the house. 'He's feeling more sociable. Aren't you, Mr T? Look who's come to see you.'

I raised a hand.

'In a couple more days he'll be fighting fit. Won't you? But probably not going to school.'

Andrea's arms, always impressively toned, hung by her sides. 'I'm so tired. My arms,' she said. 'It's been all hands to the pump and physio pretty much all day.'

'All day?'

'And night. Zoe and I have been doing it in shifts.'

Andrea's strategy of zen simplicity, of finding beauty and happiness amid strife and chaos, seemed to have reached its limits.

The notion that I had had in my mind that Sonny was a glowing hearth around which we all sang songs seemed wide of the mark. Sonny was like a family Aga, that was true, but one which Andrea and Maff were pushing up a hill. I was looking at a woman who was engaged in gruelling, repetitious round-the-clock hard work. Noble, certainly, but absolutely knackering.

The next week I fell ill with flu, and I think told a couple of people who must have mentioned it to Andrea. She rang me and asked if I wanted a soup delivery.

A day or two later I received this text:

*Hey love. How are you feeling? Delilah had an emergency appendectomy early hours Saturday morn. She became unwell*

*Friday morning and went downhill quite quickly. She's recovering well at home for a couple of weeks.*

*Hope you're getting better, Guy. Shout if you need help Sending love from me and the family xxxx*

Note the characteristic generosity of her last phrase. To offer to look after me with all she had on her hands was peak-Andrea.

## 30

## In the holidays I went skating

I became aware of the government cutting costs for people on benefits. I kept hearing about it on the radio, particularly on phone-ins. Sonny had sensitised me to many issues around disability – issues which in pre-Sonny days I carefully ignored. I heard a person say that it was impossible to get a carer on New Year's Day. A small, but significant injury.

I used to think how generously Sonny was treated by the State, but the change of care package had reduced the numbers and hours of carers. Covid, and the subsequent recession, had created relentless pressure on Andrea and Maff. When the war in Ukraine kicked off, just keeping Sonny warm during the period of energy price inflation was a challenge.

I asked Andrea about making ends meet.

'For the first time, I'm being paid carer's allowance, £69 a week,' she said, almost shamefully. 'I've never done that before. I didn't want to take it from Sonny. They tend to take it from one pot and put it in another, but I thought I have to have this money or we haven't got enough to eat. It's just one of those things,' she smiled. I could see how it hurt her pride, and told her that she was entitled to it.

Andrea grabbed our hands and leapt with us over the chasm we couldn't even look into. We were safely across but the love required to defy gravity took its toll.

I suggested I went round, hoping I could raise morale, but received this text:

*We are going to a funeral on Thursday. Boy from Sonny's class. Second one. Knew him for years.*

When I did go round, Sonny was back on the Eye-Gaze. It said 'I'm going to Liverpool, I can't wait. In the holidays I went skating.'

Andrea had loaded a number of phrases into the Eye-Gaze memory, which she said Sonny could play by looking at icons on the screen. But, remembering Anna Stubblefield's 'facilitated communication', I doubted. I thought that if his eyes went anywhere on the screen it activated the voice files, which were now spoken in a younger, more life-like tone than Hawkingese.

'That's very strange,' I said. 'Whose voice is it?'

'It's Sonny's,' said Andrea. 'He doesn't have his own.'

The machine said, 'I'm going to Liverpool, I can't wait. In the holidays I went skating.'

It was chilling hearing this disembodied voice which, I now suspected and feared, was entirely Andrea's.

'How was the skating trip?' I asked.

While she leant forward and showed me some photos, she told me she had taken Sonny in his chair and pushed him round with the other kids. I could see in the background what looked like an alarmed and angry supervisor staring at Andrea. The whole scene looked beautifully Andrea-compliant, in other words totally uncompliant.

As she stood up I saw her wince.

'What's up?' I said.

'My back's been playing up.' I knew her well enough to know that 'playing up' for Andrea meant exquisite torture to a normal person.

'He's getting big. He's growing up. He's heavy to pick up. Maff's back is bad from it too.'

## 31

## Heavy

I knew that the bedroom at the back of the house had been built because he had grown too heavy to carry up and down the stairs, and that was four years ago. There was a hoist and a sling attached to the ceiling above Sonny's bed which was attached to a rail which ran into the bathroom. I had only once briefly glimpsed Sonny dangling on the hoist when the door was ajar, and I had stepped back. That intimate part of his life was private, and keeping it that way helped him be my friend and not just subject. I hoped it dignified him, and was how I would want to be treated in such a vulnerable situation. But again, I was reviewing those thoughts. Why was I ascribing feelings and thoughts to Sonny when I had no evidence he possessed any?'

Sonny was fed the best, nourishing, tasty vegetarian (mainly) diet I had ever seen served to a child, because of course Sonny could not secretly snack or binge on confectionery or crisps, and was absolutely not overweight, but he was growing bigger. He was going to be seventeen next year. And that meant heavier. Moving him from the bed to his chair was going to get really difficult.

The problem of children with no mobility growing up and becoming heavier was, of course, not confined to Sonny. I read many accounts of its difficulties and the solutions people found for it, but the most remarkable and notorious was a child called Ashley born in the USA in 1997. She, like Sonny, could not move.

Her dad said in an interview, 'You want to be able to carry her. You start having difficulties including her in activities.' When I read that I inwardly smiled at the image of Sonny being spun around the ice-skating centre, but I knew what he meant. Ashley's parents referred to her as their 'pillow angel', which has become a well-known term for a child with a condition like Sonny.

Ashley's parents got the notion that her added size and weight were her worst enemy. They decided that a hysterectomy and a gland removal from her breasts would hold back puberty and stop her growing into a heavier and larger woman. They argued also that she would look, as a permanent child, more matched to her mental age. They also pointed out that other children have hormonal treatment to either increase or decrease their heights, which was true.

Ashley, at the age of six, had a hysterectomy and double mastectomy in a hospital in the USA.

That was quite a sentence to write, and I am sure to read. When I discovered about Ashley I never spoke to Andrea about it. There were some subjects I had learnt to keep away from: abortion, faeries being real, crystals genuinely working and the 'plandemic' being a few of them. Ashley would fall into that same category. There was no other side of the story. Andrea would not have approved.

The doctors, for some reason or another, published a paper in a medical journal about Ashley and her treatment. It sparked a bit of a firestorm. People said that mutilating a child entirely for the benefit of the parents was not acceptable. Some agitated to have the licences of the doctors revoked. The parents found themselves under a barrage of criticism but, according to what I read, also a great deal of support.

Ashley's parents' case was not helped by a woman called Anne McDonald, who had growth attenuation therapy as a severely disabled child, and at sixteen learnt to communicate (I'm not sure how, I couldn't find out), and said she wished she had been allowed to grow.

## 32

### Shark's head socks

I drove over to Frome through winter mist. The woods and hedgerows stood still, damp and cold, waiting miserably for spring. I parked on the kerb and hurried up the slope to the Thompson home almost tripping on a loose shoelace that trailed like my doubts.

Through the glass in the front door I could see Fox hurling herself at the handle and barking at the sight of me.

Andrea opened the door.

'Hello,' I said. 'How're you feeling?'

'Great!' she beamed at me.

'Have you had some good news?' I asked.

'Every day I get good news,' she replied. 'Every day. And so do you, Guy. Tea?'

And there was Sonny, in his throne, his feet pointing towards me in his shark's head socks.

She handed me a mug and said, 'You sit and chat with Sonny, I've got to sort out some stuff. Back in a minute,' and dashed off around the corner and got on the phone. 'Hiya!...'

I sat down, glanced at Sonny and then looked away out of the window at the steep terraces of the loved and neglected garden. I thought about what I had been up to all those times when I had been speaking to him. I had had chats that lasted half an hour.

To myself, and I guess as a last throw of the dice, to Sonny, I said, 'Give me a sign, Sonny, please, I beg you. Don't just bounce one back at me. Give me something I'm not expecting... please. Just give me a sign. Anything.'

I scanned his body, lying limply in the chair. One of the machines gave a beep, as it sometimes did, but I knew it was the machine and not Sonny. Right at that moment everything seemed the machine and not Sonny. I blew a lungful of air through my teeth. Talking to him was like dropping a pebble into a well and hearing nothing.

'Shit,' I said, looking down the well.

I could hear Andrea in the distance, her voice a song of positivity. I really didn't want to let her down. But all those cosy thoughts and feelings I had attributed to Sonny were no more than make-believe. The night of the Glastonbury Festival, Andrea and I could have been in the backstage bar of the Avalon stage getting caned rather than communing with Sonny, for all he knew.

## Shark's head socks

For something to do I looked at the art hanging in the lounge: a framed collage of joyful and joyous photographs of the family, the children looking young. Sonny prominently featured. A decorated graphic with the word FAMILY in the middle surrounded by positive adjectives: LOVING, HAPPY, TOGETHERNESS. The whole gallery glowed with harmony.

'Yeah! If you pick her up and take her to dance, I'll get Sam to take her for an hour till...'

I found the wide leather arm of the sofa comfy, and I looked at Sonny again.

Had I grown into the habit of not examining his expression too carefully, because it was easier for me to imagine things that way? Easier for me to impress my thoughts and words on him?

As an experiment I stared at him with steady wide eyes while I listened to the uniform breaths. Since my doubts had started over Sonny's consciousness, I had particularly noticed how, when I was in conversation with people, I picked up on their shortening or lengthening breaths. Sonny's breathing was metronomic. It was probably one of the reasons I always found him so calm, and so soothing. But it wasn't Sonny breathing. It was the ventilator. His eyes roamed the room around me, then stopped, I couldn't see what on, then moved on. He did not return my stare.

'Hello old chap,' I said, conversationally. I settled myself and watched him now softly. I breathed slowly and held my gaze firmly on his features. I communed with his face. After a couple of minutes I saw what I had glimpsed in the past but had then lost. It was a kind of emotional weather that played on his features, like passing clouds moving shadows across a hill or a shower of rain falling far out to sea.

I breathed again, deeply, and exhaled slowly. I told myself that it was okay to have doubts. Of course there would be doubts.

'I've been very worried about you,' I said to Sonny. 'You should have seen some of the stuff I've looked at. It has really made me doubt you. Made me doubt myself too, and this whole... you know... thing. Look, I even asked you to give me a sign. I know, stupid. But I've been worried that I'm just picking up from you things that I've put there, on your face, if you see what I mean.... And to be honest I'm a bit desperate...'

I closed my eyes, opened them, and Sonny was looking at me. He didn't often look at me, but he was this time.

'What do they call it?' I asked him. 'Dissonance. People describe it by saying their heart tells them one thing and their mind another. It's not quite that simple for me, but I am aware I believe things about you, like how can you put feelings and thoughts in me about the world and yourself – but they are so damned delicate I can hardly grasp them. I have tried to describe the process, but it kind of disappears as soon as I start explaining it. It's like trying to pick up sunlight. There is no language for the communication you practise, my friend!'

This was a conversation I thought I was going to have to have with Andrea, but it was to Sonny I needed to address the subject of my doubts. It felt right telling him about them.

I repeated, 'It's okay to have doubts. I realise that. Anyone would have doubts in this situation.' I paused. 'Did I just say that? Or did you?' I said. 'Did you say that?'

I smiled and reached out for his hand.

'My friend. We have departed the mechanical, chemical and biological world and arrived in the realms of the magical and mysterious.'

I smiled conspiratorially.

'It is okay to have doubts,' I repeated, adding 'But I know that you are my friend, and I am yours. Why on earth did I say I think you aren't all here, present and sentient? You are my goddam friend. We have a friendship. Don't we? If you don't have doubt, you don't have truth. Yes. You have to deal with doubt,' I added. 'What was I thinking? You are my friend. Therefore you exist. Ergo. Thank God I've worked that out.'

Andrea put her head around the corner and said, 'What have you two been chatting about?'

'We've been working something out,' I said.

'I am pleased to hear it. I don't want any arguments. What do you want to do?' she said to Sonny. 'Shall we listen to some Disney feel-good songs? Yes? I know. We can get Fox to do *The Lion King*. He loves being baby cub Mufasa.'

'This, I want to see,' I said.

Andrea leant forward and switched on the Eye-Gaze.

Sonny said, 'I'm going to Liverpool. I can't wait. In the holidays I went skating.'

She located the track from *The Lion King* on her phone, turned it up, found Fox, picked up the terrier and held him in her outstretched arm, threw back her head and wailed the opening lyrics of Circle of Life:

'Nants ingonyama bagithi baba, Sithi uhm ingonyama!'

Fox lifted her chin proudly, well-versed at playing the part of the young lion prince.

I was back to reality.

I had heard the pebble hit the water. It was just a very deep well.

## 33

### **Test results**

'We've had the results of some tests I want to tell you about,' Andrea said.

'Oh yes?' I said.

'Come round and we'll tell you,' she said. 'It's face to face news.'

'Come to me,' I said, 'bring everyone, I'll do a barbeque.'

I had been abroad, the gardener had quit to become a rock star, and the garden, which was usually clipped and closely tended, was overgrown with grasses and weeds.

Andrea took a look at it and said, 'I love the garden now you've stopped ruining it.'

Maff, Andrea and I were standing around the fire-dish in front of my house while the sausages and peppers cooked on a bed of charcoal, along with a rubber gardening glove which accidentally fell in until we smelled it and pulled it out. The children played in the undergrowth and Sonny sat beside us, wreathed in a leopard print stole.

'So, what's this news about a test?' I asked. 'I thought you already had the lost diagnosis. Did Sonny have another blood test?'

'No, we had blood tests,' Andrea said.

'...you two? Why?'

'We didn't know if it was genetic. Now we know it's genetic, we wanted to know which one of us it came from. We wanted to be informed for the children's sake, if they wanted to start their own families in the future.'

That made sense. I had never really thought about it before, but I guess they wanted to know if the Sonny gene was likely to be passed on to Finn, Talulah or Delilah, and from them to their children. It was a bit of a chilling thought. I had not really wondered about this before, though I had once said to Andrea, 'Weren't you worried you might have a second disabled child when you conceived Talulah and Deli?' And she said, 'No, not really.'

'Also,' Andrea said, 'Sonny had an MRI scan to compare it to one he had a few years ago in *2006* to look at the brain to see if there were any changes.'

I put my drink down and found a cigarette.

'Wow,' I said. 'A bit of a big moment.' I looked at them to see if I could detect which one of them had the gene, now they knew.

Maff said, 'I was worried it was going to be Andrea. I didn't want her to be burdened by it.' I absolutely believed that. That was exactly the man Maff was. He put her and Sonny and the other kids before him. Always. It was humbling to see.

Andrea said, 'I wasn't worried.' I believed that too, extraordinary as it sounded. First, Andrea, in her way, only told the truth. Second, Andrea didn't see any shame or even problem being responsible for Sonny. It would be a matter of pride for Andrea.

'So,' I said. 'Which one of you was it?'

'It actually turned out to be both of us,' Maff said.

'You both have the gene?' I said.

'Yes.'

'How unusual is it?'

'It's a very rare gene,' Andrea said. 'Very rare. I know the name of it, I'll show you the letter. It's like one in half a million people have it in the general population. If one of you have it you don't get a disabled child, but if both of you have it there is a one in four chance of having a Sonny.'

It took me a moment to take that on board. 'So, you both have it? But you didn't know?'

'No,' they said together.

'And you have four children, one of whom is Sonny,' I said. 'So that was a hell of a risk,' I said.

'Depends how you look at it,' she said.

'Both of you had this ... extremely rare genetic disorder,' I said, repeating it, almost talking to myself. 'Both of you had it, without knowing.' I shook my head in disbelief. What was I thinking? This was more than just coincidence. I had gone full-on-Andrea.

Andrea said 'When the consultant told us, I was quite blown away. I thought that's really quite beautiful in a tragic way.'

There was a gap as a cloud of gathering thoughts gusted like the smoke from the fire between us.

'Maybe,' I said, 'it was like Sonny was out there and had to bring you two together to be born into the world.'

'Yeah,' said Andrea. 'And don't forget, I was a paramedic before Sonny was born. I was equipped and ready for action and had all the knowledge to look after him all his life ...'

'.... And Maff had the strength and the patience and the love,' I said. 'The perfect couple for the job.' I turned to Sonny and said, 'I put it to you, Sonny Thompson, that you chose these parents, that you brought them together and came into their family. It was the only way you could be sure to be born and survive and be looked after. This is so weird. I seem to have turned into your mum.'

'But can't you see it's true, Guy?' Andrea said. 'How else can you explain how me and Maff are together?'

# Test results

Maff said, 'We had the blood tests because we wanted to let the children know ... if they were in a position to start a family, what they would want to do. They can now have a blood test, can ask to be tested for the gene, because it's possible to find if you are looking for it.'

I went over to slice and butter some buns. The smoke was following me.

'Finn wants the test,' Andrea said beside me.

'That's a brave move,' I said.

Finn wasn't at that barbeque, but he had been over to my house during the summer. He had stood on my lawn with his hood up and his hands deep in his pockets, fizzing with mute fury. He had an unyielding expression which scared me. It was why I had avoided him.

He was now one of the Hearthwork pirates, away from port for days at a time, marauding around festivals raising hell and canvas. Actually, when I did get to talk to him he was commendably sensitive and sensible, unlike most of that wreck-head crew. We had sat by a glowing fire in the dying light, listening to the crackle of wood and shifting logs as the smoke gusted around us.

I asked him how he dealt with the period when Sonny was in hospital for a year. 'How old were you then?' I said.

'Between six and eight. I've sort of forgotten. It's a kind of denial. Later in my life when I went past that hospital it sent me into a panic attack, flicking the trauma switch in my brain.'

'It must have been horrible,' I said.

'I've forced myself to forget.'

'That's a high-risk strategy, in my experience,' I said, 'locking bad stuff away.'

'It wasn't all bad, because I got to miss school. I hated school, and I got a lot of time on my own.'

I remembered the footsteps I used to hear upstairs when I first went round to the house in Frome. They were Finn, alone in his room for hours.

'What do you make of Sonny?' I ask.

'I love him unconditionally,' he said without hesitation, 'but it's a confusing and complicated one.'

'Can you make sense of his Eye-Gaze talk?' I asked.

'Not really. But whether it's gibberish or not, it is really important for him to have his voice.'

I had many times watched Finn's tenderness with his brother, arranging a scarf here, re-positioning his cap, checking if he wanted more suction, adjusting his chair so he could see some action.

'My social skills were terrible because I couldn't play with Sonny,' Finn admitted. 'I used to fight people and get angry because I didn't know how kids worked. And the way some people reacted to Sonny – I had to learn not to be offended at other people's ignorance. Am I angry? Oh yeah. I am angry at the world and at people.'

But an hour after he said that I watched him patiently and lovingly load Sonny into the Zombie Outbreak Response Vehicle, and give me such a warm and friendly hug goodbye. He was nineteen, his life ahead of him; he was on his journey out of the nest and away from Sonny, which would surely be a relief for him.

For Andrea and Maff the same journey was not a possibility. Thank god their marriage seemed so strong.

'How do you maintain your marriage so successfully?' I asked.

'We both came from broken homes, and we both didn't want to repeat that,' Maff said.

'We come across a problem, we work it out.'

'You make it sound very easy,' I said.

'We have to communicate,' Andrea said. 'We just have to.'

Maff added, 'We know how it would be for one of us on our own.'

That created a rueful silence, broken by Andrea saying, 'It needs to be teamwork.' To Maff, she said, 'You're not allowed to die. Okay?' To me, she said, 'We have this competition with each other over who's going to die first.'

But I didn't point out that it is likely that Sonny would die before them. They were spared the agony of parents of disabled children who worry about who will protect their children after they die.

'Sonny's friend died. We were the only parents from school at the funeral,' said Andrea. 'We had to go, and Sonny had to go. They had been friends for years.'

## 34

### Fixture

I was off to a major Premier League fixture to watch the team I loved from a seat right beside the pitch. The van failed its MOT the day before we were meant to leave, but Andrea knew of a charity who could help out. They found a replacement vehicle while Sonny's was being fixed. The new van was smaller than the Zombie Outbreak Response Vehicle and lacked a back seat, though with a bit of persuasion Maff got them to fit one.

I called the hotel and reserved the same set of rooms, and Andrea spoke to Air Liquide and organised the portable oxygen cylinders and an oxygen concentrator to be waiting at the hotel.

Carers Zoe and Nula were alerted, booked, and given train tickets so they could be at the hotel when we arrived in Liverpool on Friday afternoon.

The evening before we were due to leave I received some bad news. A movie project I was working on for Netflix was axed. It had been in development for a year, and it looked like being a big break – as well as earner – for me. I was upset when I read the email, sitting at my kitchen table in front of a bowl of closed tulips. My agent tried to soften the blow by saying many other writers were in the same boat as me. But it didn't help.

When I arrived at the house in Frome Sonny was in front of the Eye-Gaze screen surrounded by chaos. I had missed him and his impenetrable weird ways, and I was ashamed that I had so fully doubted him. I particularly wanted to share the Netflix rejection with him. That, he would understand. I wanted to tell him about it, like I did in the early days, and he would understand and dispense, in his magical way, solace and comfort. What better person to share news of a setback with than Sonny Thompson, the master of the art of overcoming obstacles?

Sonny emanated a compassion that made life soothing. And I was not concerned about doubting him. Nobody was more forgiving than Sonny. He radiated it. Then I remembered Radiator Peach. He couldn't use words, or signs. He could only radiate. Was that what he was telling us when he said Radiator Peach?

'It's so daunting, there's so much to think of,' Andrea said as Fox bolted around the room filled with boxes, cylinders and suitcases.

'I can't find the Eye-Gaze bag,' she said, budging boxes towards the door. They were always lugging equipment.

'That's his suction face,' Andrea said, looking around for the box of long straws.

'Want want want stop wanting want to stop wanting wanting to stop seeing,' Sonny said.

'I feel you want to turn it off?' said Andrea.

'Is he after the TV?' I asked.

'He's after his diary,' said Andrea, and touched the screen a few times until Sonny said, 'We went to Sherbourne Zoo. I went to the cinema with my mum. I loved being pushed really fast and doing skids on the ice.'

'I never knew you went to the cinema,' I said, then realised it would be a perfect outing because he was always silent.

'Cinema's great,' said Andrea. 'We get cheap tickets with the CEA card and two carers go in for free.'

'We went to Sherbourne Zoo,' Sonny's machine said.

Andrea appeared with a huge syringe full of orange liquid. She attached it to the tube that disappeared under Sonny's shirt and pressed home the plunger. With her other hand, she held his hand.

'Will you give him breakfast?' She handed me a bowl of blended banana and oat milk and another large syringe. I placed the end into the goo and pulled back the plunger, filling the syringe. Then I reached under his shirt and found the tube attached to the stent and fixed the syringe into the tube and tightened the little ribbed wheel. Then I pressed my thumb down and watched the banana shoot round the tube and disappear into Sonny. I had never fed him before. It definitely felt like feeding a child, yet there was absolutely no mess. And of course Sonny couldn't taste it, or possibly even smell it. The jury was out on that one. He had no say on the speed I fed him, but I tried to calculate it at the speed I would eat. He made a few gurgles. One of the machines started beeping quietly.

'What's that?' I asked.

'Why are you beeping, Sonny?' Andrea put down a box and looked at the machines on the back of the chair. 'I BPE. Whatever that means. Could be a small blockage, or the ventilator has slowed down or he needs a suction.'

The beeping stopped on its own accord. 'That's that sorted,' she laughed. 'There's a really good children's hospital in Liverpool if we forget anything.' Of course, I remembered, Sonny was only ever one battery away from death.

Then she said, as if commenting on the warm weather, 'Did I tell you Sonny has to have a pacemaker? Every year they do a cardiac twenty-four-hour tape. A sleep study. It's a twenty-four-hour tape from a heart monitor. Anyway, they want to fit a pacemaker.'

'Bloody hell, isn't that a bit of a major thing?' I said.

'The consultant wants a twelve-day test to be sure. But Sonny has been through so much recently with his chest. And you know the letter says with Sonny's autism it will be difficult. But Sonny doesn't have the markers for autism.'

Last minute checks were going on.

'Which hat do you want? This one or this one?' Andrea stood in front of the prince on his throne. 'This one? This one? This one, this one. Okay we'll take them both.'

We wheeled Sonny out and up the ramp into the van. Maff secured Sonny's chair to the floor of the van with straps and hooks. Then he ran through the final check for all the chargers – vent chargers, phone chargers. Checked both chairs, stents, feeding tubes. He was so careful.

## 35

**Sprinkles and whipped cream**

In Starbucks, at a service station on the motorway, Andrea bought Sonny a hot chocolate with sprinkles and whipped cream. While they got comfortable at a table in the middle of the restaurant – no table hidden away at the back for Andrea – I got the drinks and received a smile of real warmth from the barista, entirely on account of my association with Sonny.

'He's wet,' said Andrea. 'Is there a disabled change? He needed changing; that was what he was shouting about.' Sonny, of course, had not made a noise beyond an involuntary gurgle, but Andrea we agreed, somehow knew.

There wasn't a disabled changing room at the service station. I wasn't certain what one would look like. The horse-box disabled toilet would obviously not be any good. He had to be laid down and changed like an infant. I didn't like writing that sentence, let alone contemplating the act because it was humiliating for Sonny. In the end they did it on some towels in the back on the van with me standing facing away with my arms crossed, warning people away. When it was over, Andrea said, 'Sorry about that, Sonny.'

Andrea was at the wheel. She used to drive ambulances and you could tell. Fast and safe. If she saw three vehicles side by side on the motorway she'd shake her head, tut, and say 'Three in a bed.' Maff was behind, suctioning Sonny and holding his hand. In this new bus Sonny could see out the front window, but his stare was inscrutable.

'He's excited. You're excited, aren't you?' said Andrea.

I hadn't been to Liverpool for ten years, and instead of approaching it as I remembered – through miles of inadequate housing and scrofulous streets – we passed huge retail parks with well-filled car parks and cavernous restaurants.

The hotel in Liverpool was downtown and up-market. City centre parking? In the van with the magic windscreen sticker we drew up on the double yellow right outside the revolving glass door with total impunity. Zoe and Nuala were waiting for us on the pavement and gave us a hand carrying in the boxes, which I noticed started filling up the refined space around the reception desk. The neat trim man on duty looked into his screen as Maff appeared out of the lift with Sonny, whose chair with all its flashing lights, tubes and wires looked at odds with the hyper elegant space. While I checked us in, Maff essayed a quick bit of physio and a suction.

## 36

## **XXXXL**

On match day morning the Liverpool Football tribe, or part of it, started assembling in the hotel lobby.

I was anxious. Andrea was anxious. 'He's a bit chesty,' she said, and ordered Sonny a full English. I hadn't managed to get a ticket for Andrea as Sonny's ticket came with just two carer seats, so she wasn't going to see the game.

A family sat on sofas close to us, the adolescent children frozen by Sonny's presence. Finn had once told me that he had a death stare he gave in such situations, but I just looked away. I didn't feel they were malicious, I thought they were scared and uneducated. Sonny had changed my attitudes to disabled people, who I now did not live in fear of contagion from.

At the tables on the other side, guests were speaking foreign languages. Most of the men and some of the women wore Liverpool shirts. I watched a man wearing an XXXXL Milner shirt destroy the six sausages, two fried eggs, eight rashers of bacon and a pyramid of baked beans from the buffet.

The pavement outside the hotel was thick with people wearing Liverpool strip. We exchanged encouraging smiles as we faced the sternest and most important test of the season: Manchester United, at home.

It was a must-win match for both teams, and a must-see match for the *700* million people watching on TV around the globe. To put that into context, the Super Bowl had an audience of *112* million.

The fixture was always brutal and tight. *1-0*, *1-1*, *2-1*. These were scores of this game over the years. And as both sides had some of the highest paid footballers on the planet, the feeling was that this time things would be no different. We were all just praying we wouldn't lose.

Swathed in his club scarf, with his red cap on his head, we loaded Sonny onto the ramp and into the van. Andrea was going to drop us off and pick us up later.

'Can you please promise me when you are in the game you won't ignore him,' she said.

'Of course not. We are right beside him,' Maff and I chorused.

'What happens if the suction machine packs in during the match?'

'We'll plug it in in the bar or Jürgen's office,' Maff said. Jürgen Klopp was the manager of Liverpool.

Andrea nudged the van through the crowd that filled the road, using her parking superpower to draw up imperiously on another double yellow. The stadium reared over us, angular, ugly and red. Maff and I went about our business. We opened the van doors and brought Sonny down to earth on the tail lift.

We aimed for the club shop, a modern warehouse rammed full of merchandise and fans. Customers turned to see us manoeuvring Sonny between the racks of shirts and shorts and scarves and all the other garments you could squeeze a Liverpool Football Club logo on.

A woman with a baseball cap with a sparkly peak stood staring at Andrea who said, standing in front of about six different shirt designs, 'Which strip do you want? Away or home? This one or this one? Do I need to find a green one? This one? This one? No.'

I now knew she could have said yes without any of us noticing. But Andrea was on her mission. She disappeared and returned with more garments.

'Black? Yellow? Yellow!!!'

A shop assistant then took us directly to the front of a fifty-person queue and checked us out, opening a special door at the back of the shop which led straight on to the forecourt of the stadium. We said goodbye to Andrea and pushed forward into the people gathering at the turnstiles to get in.

A man passed us, turned to Sonny and said, 'Bring us luck, pal.'

He might not be able to say exactly which shirt he wanted, but everybody could feel Sonny radiate.

## 37

### **Touchline village**

We couldn't go through a turnstile with Sonny. If we had tried, god knows what would have come out the other side. We were admitted through a wide door up a concrete ramp which, after a couple of turns, led straight out into the stadium at pitch level.

The scent of turf was always a breath-taking moment at a Premier League stadium, whatever level I came in on. The flawless green baize of the pitch with its bright white lines sped my heartbeat. Something so often seen, and only ever on a screen, was now right in front of me. Adrenalin supercharged the air. Coming in at ground level, the sound of the boots on the ball as the teams warmed up was percussively close. You could hear the players – our gods – talking to each other and laughing. Mohammed Salah, the Egyptian King, only ever a tiny figure on a TV screen, was just feet away from Sonny, Maff and me.

Around and behind us the stadium filled. The section to our right was reserved for the Manchester United supporters. They were conducted in as a group to prevent individuals getting caught in a crowd of Liverpool fans and creating friction. They were in good voice. We had a classic encounter on our hands.

A steward walked towards us. 'Hiya chuck, would you be Sonny Thompson?' she said, and led us to our seats.

The supporters in wheelchairs were parked on a wide concrete strip marked out with numbered yellow rectangles. It turned out that nearly all of these people, and there were about forty in number, were friends. As season ticket holders, they and their carers met every fortnight on this spot to watch the team play. A few spaces were reserved for non-season-ticket holders, and we took our position just to the side of the goal in one of these: Sonny in the square and Maff and me in flip-down seats behind.

With the stadium full, and the players back in the changing room for their final preparations, the crowd, all 54,000 of them - minus the United supporters – started to sing the Liverpool Football Club anthem.

'When you walk through a storm,' the ranks sang, 'hold your head up high, and don't be afraid of the dark. At the end of a storm there's a golden sky, and the sweet silver song of a lark.' A huge collective breath was drawn, then they bellowed 'Walk on, through the wind! Walk on, through the rain! Though your dreams be tossed and blown, walk on with hope in your heart and you'll never walk alone, you'll never walk alone!'

It was almost unbearable to sing it standing beside Sonny.

After the anthem, Maff held Sonny's hand while he took him through the match programme, page by page.

When the woman in the wheelchair to my left let her glasses fall off her lap I was astonished to see her lean down and pick them up. I soon saw that no one in the disabled area was as limited as Sonny.

The match started; the crowd bristled at a foul. Then it roared with encouragement and booed at a mistake. We were part of a huge organic entity. I looked at Sonny. I had imagined that he would pick up on the immense power of the emotion in the air around him.

A strike on goal just went wide, Maff said, 'Oh yes,' and gave Sonny a quick suction.

Then, twenty feet in front of us, Liverpool's Cody Gakpo, the club's new signing, scored a goal and the place went wild. Maff jumped up and down and turned to kiss Sonny. We were one nil up against United. We had heard and seen, unamplified, the ball thump into the bulging net right in front of us, with people all over the world watching on TV.

Could we survive to half-time without conceding a goal? The atmosphere in the stadium shifted from triumph to anxiety. Then, two minutes later, Darwin Núñez, our Uruguayan striker, glanced the ball into the net to make it *2-0*. Cheers, laughter, smiles and unbounded happiness all around. It was impossible not to feel the thrill.

The husband of the lady who dropped her glasses returned from a visit to the bar with a cup of juice for his wife.

'Did you miss the goals?' someone asked.

As he gave the drink to his wife he grinned ruefully and said to me, 'That's what caring's about.'

'Thank you, love,' she said.

Maff took a photo of Sonny in front of the bouncing crowd and said, 'Gonna send this one to Rolfy.' Rolfy was Maff's best friend, a man I had never met but knew adored Sonny.

Half-time gave us an opportunity to give Sonny another suction and check the batteries. Around me, the village started exchanging gossip and talking about the match and season. There was a rumour going round that the new owners, a bunch of Americans, wanted to rebuild the seating, shunting the disabled section away from the pitch to an upper tier.

## 38

## Second half

When play restarted, the fans around us picked on the carer who had been getting his wife a drink when the goals were scored. 'Get out of here! Go on! We need more goals.'

Liverpool were now attacking the far goal, and it was harder to see what was going on, but a roar from the crowd and a cluster of players in wild celebration told us we had a third. Nobody could really believe it. We were 3-0 up against United. It was almost unprecedented. Jubilation and hallelujahs all around. Ten minutes later we scored a fourth, tucked away by Mohammed Salah.

The stadium rang with his chant:

*Mo salah la la la la Mo Salah la la la la*

*If he's good enough for me he's good enough for you*

*If he scores another few*

*Then I'll be Muslim too.*

*Sitting in a mosque that's where I want to be*

And suddenly we were *4-0* up, courtesy of the Egyptian King again. Absolute ecstasy, writ over fifty thousand faces. Glancing around the supporters on the terrace, I saw that the woman to my left, the one who had been able to reach down and pick up her glasses, had taken an interest in Sonny. She had straight brown hair, cut short, a sharp nose and raking eyes when she twisted her neck to check out Sonny. She kept looking away and then back at him. With so much going on about us, I expect she thought nobody could see her staring.    I    imagined she was wondering what was going on with him. She was trying to work out the enigma that was Sonny Thompson. Swathed in Liverpool Football club merchandise he was a teenager watching his football team thrash their greatest opponents right under his nose, but was exhibiting absolutely no emotion.

She stared at Sonny's stillness.

To her, he was making no attempts at communication. Everybody was cheering, singing, pointing, and booing, fully animated, with the exception of Sonny, and, to be fair, the Manchester United supporters penned to my right who were growing stiff in their pain and fury. Though at *6-0* they too became animated, hurling javelin insults at their own players.

When a steward in a yellow tabard walked in front of us a supporter leapt up from his wheelchair and screamed '*Sit down!*'

The woman still watched Sonny. She looked away at the play, and looked back.

I thought she was saying to herself, there's nothing going on in there. That annoyed me. And I realised that through a process of reverse engineering my resentment was further proof of Sonny's presence. I wanted to tap her on the shoulder and explain that Sonny was feeling the match, the stadium full of supporters, and even the score. Maybe he didn't feel the precise number of goals, but he knew it was the kind of victory that would be remembered and talked about for many years ahead.

Had I spoken to her, I would have said to her come close to Sonny; you too can feel his presence.

Maff grinned and punched the air. I had lost interest in the match but was vaguely aware of Liverpool scoring a seventh goal. I was just staring at Sonny with such intensity a high-pitched whine rang in my ears blocking out the background cacophony of that extraordinary afternoon.

This single, piercing note keening in my ears preceded a truth: what was going on inside Sonny was by no means the only extraordinary thing about this young man. Another of his great gifts to me, his family, friends and the world, was what went on around him, and what effect he had on us all. And events that day conspired to illustrate this gloriously.

Later, it was generally agreed in the Thompson household that it was Sonny's presence at Anfield stadium which occasioned the historic seven goal win. To Andrea, it was just obvious and indisputable. Given the chance, in the next fixture, she would have played Sonny up front.

When the full-time whistle blew people were clambering over the seats to hug each other. Maff jumped up and down in the arms of a stranger. People patted Sonny and shook his hand. A woman hugged him.

Normal service resumed. The noise of the crowd returned. I was amongst thousands of happy people beaming with joy, with Sonny sitting there amongst this mayhem with an expression of total unperturbability. But life was like this for Sonny. Beautiful things, miraculous things, occurred around him every day. It may well have been that as far as he was concerned, nothing extraordinary had happened that afternoon.

The crowd sang out again.

The Manchester United supporters stood with their arms folded, glaring with fury. I saw two with tears running down their faces.

We hadn't suctioned Sonny since 3-0, so we quickly attended to that and checked the batteries. All good. All brilliant. Two of the supporters in the front row shouted, 'You better bring that lad back next week.'

I thought to myself, and I said to Sonny, 'What a miraculous afternoon.' Because I was talking to him again. We were back on terms. And I knew without doubt whose good it was for: mine.

## 39

## **Sapling**

Sonny was a sapling, planted by Andrea and Maff, which over the seasons they had loved and tended. Each leaf that unfurled gave them hope that their little tree would grow, and one day blossom, bear fruit, throw out branches, give shade and create its own saplings.

But the Sonny sapling had not thrived, grown tall and thrown out branches. Andrea still painstakingly watered, fed and talked to the tree, but only a few leaves appeared. Sometimes a leaf dropped off, or a bud dried and died. Everybody, me included, stared at the sapling, and prayed for spring to bring forth blossom. We implored the branches and twigs to come to life and bear fruit. Our prayers were not fully answered, at least not in the way we hoped.

What we failed to see, as we stared at the branches and tried to will another bud to form, was that on the ground around the tree, where Andrea had watered the earth and Maff had worked fertiliser into the dirt, the seeds of other plants had settled, germinated, and taken root. All around us, grasses of different heights, textures and colours had sprouted and created a meadow, and in that meadow wild flowers of many colours and shapes took root and thrived.

Because I had spent all my time staring at the tree with two leaves on it, praying that one wouldn't drop off, I had not noticed that I was standing in Sonny's garden.

All the people who spent time around Sonny came into flower and bloomed with kindness and compassion. His cognitive ability was irrelevant. He gave us all great solace. I had asked myself the day before, what was the point of telling him about my woes? What was the point of talking to him about the Netflix failure? But there was every point. His withheld or non-existent powers of reaction and judgement made him perfect to commune with on sensitive subjects. His epic silence, his refusal or inability to ever have an opinion or make a statement made him the perfect friend and the finest company. That was why I had missed him.

It was true that there were not monuments or cathedrals rising up out of the landscape of Sonny's life, but the view was certainly not clear all the way to the horizon. I just had to lower my gaze and look more closely. Then I saw the flowers and the butterflies of the plain, I heard the trickle of a stream, the hum of bees and the songs of the birds. Everything was coming into flower every day. Sonny's landscape was busy with love, beauty and small divine moments.

Andrea had created a rich meadow, which would never have flowered and never have flourished had she not tended Sonny's tree.

When people think that the best thing for this world would be that when Sonny goes to sleep tonight he doesn't wake up in the morning, they overlook the fact that regardless of the weary trope that a person left the world a better place, the phrase would never be more owned by anybody with more force than Sonny Thompson. And who could wish harm on Sonny? His tree gave hope, and fruit, to us all, it being a peach tree.

## 40

**Barnsey**

When we left the brightness of the floodlit stadium, we found ourselves in the dark under a shower of silver rain slanting in the streetlights. A complicated, purposeful crowd swirled around us, catching us in its currents, like a river of people in spate. Nipping into a pub was out of the question, we could see the customers squeezed at the doors and hear the songs of glory being sung inside. We had agreed to meet Andrea where she dropped us off outside the club shop, but the road had been closed to all vehicles.

We set off with Maff pushing Sonny down the hill through oncoming people.

Maff said, 'Did that really happen?'

Despite the dire weather and a number of misunderstandings with Andrea about where to meet, meaning we had to walk at least two miles, we were joyous and happy. Andrea wasn't.

'Let's get back to the hotel and buy you a big Bloody Mary,' I suggested as she patiently operated the ramp, checked it for safety and rolled Sonny into the truck.

We made it back to the hotel, got to the reception area and Maff remembered he had left his programme in the van. He wanted to savour it. Andrea had nipped up to change, and I went over to the bar to order some drinks leaving Sonny alone in the middle of reception. It was an unusual thing to do, but I knew I would only be twenty paces away from him at the bar, with an eye on him all the time. I turned to the bartender and ordered a couple of beers and a Bloody Mary. When I looked back I saw that Sonny was still in place.

With his beeping instruments and flashing lights he looked like an astronaut recently arrived from another planet.

I waved at him even though I knew he couldn't see me, or respond, but I did it to show anyone watching that he was not alone. I was proud to be his friend. While I watched the bartender pour my drink I thought about how Sonny had opened my heart, and how good it felt.

Behind Sonny, the revolving door paddled a faintly familiar figure into the hotel. The man, in his sixties, wore jeans and a brown leather coat. Then I recognised who it was: it was John Barnes, the legendary Liverpool player who Maff had idolised from childhood.

I watched John Barnes look around and notice Sonny sitting in front of him, and was about to launch myself away from the bar to intervene when I hesitated, to see what would happen. John Barnes approached Sonny with a smile on his broad, handsome face, leaning over to say something in his ear. I needed to go and explain that Sonny couldn't talk, or did I?

The matter was settled when Maff came through the spinning door to see Sonny in the middle of reception with a total stranger. I enjoyed seeing the precise moment Maff recognised John Barnes. Rocked back on his heels, he stared at the man, until Barnes put out his hand and introduced himself.

The lift doors opened and Andrea stepped out. When she got to Maff and Sonny, and was introduced to John Barnes, she let out a peal of laughter that filled the bar. Maff fumbled for his phone and John Barnes posed for a picture beside Sonny. I saw the photo later: Maff's hand had been shaking so much and he forgotten to turn on the flash so it was a murky blur. But it didn't matter. Nothing could take that moment from them.

## 41

### The beautiful game

John Barnes went on his way and we gathered around a table. Andrea had her Bloody Mary, and Sonny a freshly squeezed orange juice. Andrea went to sit beside him, to enjoy his excitement. He lived in a box room at the back of the house in Frome, Somerset, and a van to and from his school. Here he was in the middle of a triumphant night on the town. Andrea snaked her arm around his and interlinked her fingers with him.

It was always comforting to hold Sonny's hand and stroke his skin. Making you feel good about yourself was a core talent. It was Friday night and everybody was out in the lobby bar: knots of girls in micro dresses and cantilevered cleavages squired by men with natty suits and beringed fingers. Sonny was sixteen years old and scoping out the women on a Friday night, and his mother was holding his hand.

I said, 'Move Sonny so he can see the punters.'

In his new position, I imagined him checking out the women of Liverpool arriving for their Friday night revels.

'That's better,' I said, and added, 'Hey Andrea, there are some seriously hot women in range. I don't think sixteen-year-old boys would really want to hold their mum's hand in this situation.'

She slid her hand out from his and moved her chair.

We all looked at Sonny in this new light, in his new persona: Sonny the smooth player out on the town.

The waiter was summoned, and he stood there while Andrea read the entire menu to Sonny. Every word of it. After which she said, 'He wants fish.'

It may have been make-believe, but it was a chance for us all to be imaginative, generous, kind and warm. Under Andrea's supervision, we had all created an astonishing bubble to dwell in, safely and enjoyably. We were in a drama, but it was a beautiful creation, and I was proud, not ashamed, to be part of it. To be that close to Sonny, Andrea and Maff was to feel the glow of a thrilling combination of compassion, love and extreme parenting.

All that time I had spent in Sonny's company, talking to him, or including him in the conversation, had not been wasted. When I spent the night of the Glastonbury Festival with him and Andrea, I was being my most generous, my most selfless, loving, patient and kind self. And it was Sonny who drew that out of me.

All the time I had been asking if Sonny was all there, but the question I should have been asking was, was I all there? Was I only going to love him if he talked or moved or said the word 'Guy'? My love was much greater if he gave me no sign and I stayed solid by his side.

## 42

## **The beginning**

When I left my room the next morning, battling through a hangover with an espresso martini of a headache, I weaved along the corridor to knock on Sonny's door. Zoe and Nuala had already left to catch their train. Maff and Andrea were making sounds but not words as they loaded up the boxes and bags, grunting, huffing, sighing, with a few low moans.

Later, I thought I remembered seeing the batteries plugged into a socket by the bedside table. But I didn't think anything of it. Because we weren't looking for them then.

The goodbyes at reception and in the restaurant were joyous, heartfelt and, in my case, teary. Everybody remembered Sonny, of course, and all adored him; he just had that effect on the staff, who came up to say goodbye and wish him well.

The way Maff triple-checked Sonny's chair moorings in the back of the van was absolutely love in action. With Sonny secured, the bags and boxes were thrown pell-mell around him as we just wanted to get home.

# The beginning

Conversation was not lively on the drive south, first through the suburbs of Liverpool and then onto the M6 under dark cloud, through the dour dimness of an early dusk and heavy rain. The wipers did their work but the traffic was sludgy, often bringing us slowly to a halt. We sat motionless for at least ten minutes, thirty miles north of Birmingham and the Spaghetti Junction.

It was then, while we were stationary in the middle lane, with vans, trucks and cars all around us, bumper to bumper, that the beeping on Sonny's ventilator battery struck up.

Beep. Beep.

Maff left his seat and started to go through the bags. He usually moved so quickly and efficiently, but the combination of a hangover and the chaos of the van slowed him down. Andrea didn't turn round. She always watched the road ahead.

Maff found a battery, looked at it and put it back down because it was uncharged.

'Try the black suitcase,' Andrea said.

Maff opened it with a click and emptied it all over the floor of the van. There was definitely no clunk of a battery falling out of the clothes.

I said, 'How much time do we have?'

Maff said 'About seven minutes.'

Andrea said, 'How far to the next service station?'

Maff opened his phone, scrolled, and said 'Frankley, twenty-three miles,' and went back through the boxes, cases and side pockets on both chairs.

I thought, we need a blue flashing light and a siren. I also thought: this is your fault, Guy, as the trip was your idea, and staying up drinking late was also my idea. I did what I often did when I felt fear rising, I reached for Sonny's soft, reassuring hand.

'Who packed them?' Andrea said.

'I don't know,' Maff replied. 'I thought Zoe or Nuala had.'

'Shit,' Andrea said.

The beeping became a constant tone.

'Fuuuuck,' said Maff.

I heard the ventilator change tone as it ran down the power. I opened the window because I thought I was going to be sick.

## 43

## Secret place

I closed my eyes and found myself walking down a dark passageway into a sealed off secret place where Sonny was not going to die in the back of a van on the M6. I could hear Maff turning everything over behind me. I thought, ah that was why we had the fairytale day yesterday. It was a flowering before the petals fell.

When I opened my eyes, Andrea was looking back at Maff and Sonny.

'Don't worry, Sonny,' she said. 'Everything's going to be okay.'

Maff stopped moving and said 'Aah.' Then I saw him holding a battery and clipping it onto the ventilator. The beeping ceased. Oh wonderful silence. And the gentle rhythm of the ventilator started.

Andrea looked ahead, her faeries-exist-and-magic-is-real smile on her face.

'It was in my coat pocket,' Maff said.

'All right, Mr T?' Andrea said.

I said, 'Christ.'

Andrea said, 'That's the thing about Sonny. He always defies predictions. He's my survivor. Aren't you?' She sunk the clutch, put the van into first and we moved forward again, down the long road ahead to home.

## Acknowledgements

This book is not mine alone. I must share the credit with Andrea and Maff Thompson who let me into their home and introduced me to their son Sonny. Always generous, trusting, kind and insightful, they helped me understand and feel what was in front of me. They censored nothing I wrote, nor took any payment (which is why if you want to help, there are details of a GoFundMe page below).

Sonny's aside, the stories of the people in this book I culled from internet forums, documentaries, medical textbooks, and personal contacts. My main background source was the phenomenal Far from the Tree, written by Andrew Solomon. If you have any interest in children who are different, I strongly recommend you read this awesome, informative and inspirational book.

Sonny's Go Fund Me page is to be found at:

https://gofund.me/*23a17ea71*

www.ingramcontent.com/pod-product-compliance
Lightning Source LLC
LaVergne TN
LVHW041800060526
838201LV00046B/1069